Gynecologic nursing

If our schools turn out their pupils in that attitude of mind which is conducive to good judgment in any department of affairs in which the pupils are placed, they have done more than if they sent out their pupils possessed merely of vast stores of information or high degrees of skill in specialized branches.

John Dewey

Gynecologic nursing

**A textbook concerning nursing through an understanding
of the patients themselves and their gynecologic problems**

John I. Brewer, M.D., Ph.D.

*Professor of Obstetrics and Gynecology, Northwestern
University Medical School, and Chief of Obstetrics and Gynecology,
Passavant Memorial Hospital, Chicago, Illinois*

Doris M. Molbo, R.N., Ph.B.

*Associate Director of Nursing Research, Hartford
Hyperbaric Unit, Lutheran General Hospital,
Park Ridge, Illinois*

Albert B. Gerbie, M.D.

*Assistant Professor of Obstetrics and Gynecology,
Northwestern University Medical School, and Attending
Obstetrician and Gynecologist, Passavant Memorial
Hospital, Chicago, Illinois*

The C. V. Mosby Company

Saint Louis   1966

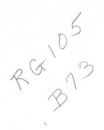

Preface

Everyone feels safe and in control when factual answers can be given to questions, and when rules and procedures can prescribe the dimensions of a theoretical subject or of an individual. Yet there are few definite answers in life. Even the respected field of scientific inquiry has had to change some of the scientific "facts" or answers about atoms and chromosomes which were once accepted, taught, and learned in schools a few years ago. Within the applied science of medicine, many of the "rules" from postoperative care to infant feeding schedules have been drastically changed within that time period. Interestingly, within the same period, a restored appreciation of the principles of medical and surgical asepsis has arisen after the early antibiotic era of overconfident disdain. Answers sometimes imply complete knowledge or satisfactory solution of the problem. They may discourage further quests or imply a static state or status quo.

A nurse asks questions and seeks answers for guidance and direction. Yet within her professional environment, she deals with ever-changing situations and ever-changing individuals within those situations. It should be no surprise then that answers are ever-changing. Although many facets of hospital life are regulated by means of administrative edict, no one's life is static—neither the patient's, her family's, nor the nurse's. No individual is the person today that he or she was yesterday, and each individual will be different tomorrow. Probably this is observed nowhere as vividly as in the daily changing picture of the postoperative patient. This book is written, therefore, with full recognition that every nurse and every individual with whom that nurse reacts will communicate, make decisions, and act within ever-changing environments, situations, and personal experiences.

This book is also written in the belief that knowledge is both objective and subjective. That is, objective information can be given in many areas; how this objective information is integrated and utilized makes it personalized or subjective. The ways in which it is interpreted and used are, therefore, affected by the kinds and complexities of past experiences, through which all new knowledge is interpreted. The ways in which knowledge is interpreted and used are also affected by the congruence (likeness) or the incongruence (conflict) of the knowledge with the present situation or action. This means that what a nurse feels about life and disease or about time and activity will influence her decisions and experiences as she faces an acute emergency, a geriatric patient, an "uneventful" postoperative patient, or a dying patient. A student's values influence her nursing knowledge and her nursing interactions with her patients or instructors, who may share her values or may not. Therefore, in ever-changing situations, and in the presence of dynamic interpersonal relationships, knowledge is more than objective facts, procedures, and do's and don't's. If new concepts are to be more than intellectualization, they must become a part of the learner and be internalized, tested, and experienced by her.

Skills in the nursing of a patient can be learned nowhere but at the bedside, in the presence of the patient and the student's instructor. This indicates the importance of the most sensitive and skilled instructor for the clinical area, as she provides the instruction and/or model of nursing by using subjective knowledge. As Sir William Osler has said, "To study the phenomena of disease without books is to sail an uncharted sea; while to study books without patients is not to go to sea at all."

It is the purpose of this book to provide some guides for the uncharted seas of human relationships of nurse and patient. Even as each sea voyage is different and unique from the last, each voyage of personal interaction requires new communications, perceptions, and interpretations. It means new decisions for differing situations in unique combination and calls forth memory of past experience, discrimination of differences, a solving of the inherent problems, and an evaluation of the course finally taken.

Within this book many questions will be raised and many problems of both patient and nurse in the gynecologic patient-nurse relationship will be exposed. This is not a "how-to" book and it provides no pat answers. It is offered with the hope that the guides herein presented will stimulate the young nurse to enter many new areas of questioning as she interacts with each new patient, will foster subjective integration and synthesis of knowledge within the experiential patient situation, and will quicken the young student's quests into the many related and supporting disciplines to nursing. To entice this quest, a varied bibliography of professional writings has been introduced. Current and typical patient readings have been included for evaluation, as well as pamphlets which may be obtained for patient use.

John I. Brewer
Doris M. Molbo
Albert B. Gerbie

Contents

Chapter 4

The postoperative patient, 42

Chapter 5

The adolescent patient, 67

Chapter 6

The mature patient, 88

Gynecologic nursing

Chapter 1

The essence of nursing

Nursing is never a passive action. When nursing exists, the action is nurture in some form, and the recipient is a patient or the patient's family. Professional nursing exists when it involves an interdisciplinary effort of the helping professions and when the peculiar knowledge and sensitivity of a nurse enable her to care for a hitherto strange human being in such a way that the healing process is sustained or actually enhanced. Sometimes this nurture may only mean supporting the bowed head and the trembling hands. If a patient or her family are not nourished, nursing is absent, even though a "nurse" may be present physically.

The sole nursing emphasis for some nurses has been the completion of a procedure, the enactment of the doctor's order, or "doing" something *to* the patient. She has not been involved in the healing regimen.

Recent reemphasis of the patient as an individual has made it a necessity to understand the underlying principles of the procedures, doctor's orders, and disease entity. Fulfillment of nursing care requires inductive and deductive thinking or problem solving to "individualize" the therapy for each patient. Since this involves perceptions, decisions, and judgments on the part of the nurse, she experiences participation in the healing regimen. Her concentration is on "doing *for*" the patient. As she formulates her nursing diagnosis, she may feel a certain partnership with the medical staff or an autonomy of her own within the healing process. Even "little doctor" stirrings may be present.

"Doing to" involves hands. "Doing for" involves intellect or head. Neither is minimized; both are essential, but they are not enough.

With few exceptions, nursing has seemed to ignore the environment and the patient, the environment and the nurse, and therefore the effect of one on another. Because nurses interact with patients 24 hours a day, they are able to evaluate the patient's environment, to know the patient's reactions to it, and to transmit this information to others involved with her care. That they often do not indicates their lack of awareness of human dynamics and of their role of nurture to the patient.

An altered physical or psychologic environment changes perceptions and communication patterns. This is often not emphasized in nurse-patient relationships. Since all personal interactions have potential beneficial or detrimental effects, nursing interactions can be said to have either beneficial or detrimental effects on all patients and ultimately on the healing process. Nursing emphasis with this focus is necessarily an interdisciplinary one or one that recognizes the imperativeness of open communication, trust, and goodwill between all involved—the helping professions, the patient, and her family. The nurse's function then is to interact *with* all involved and to cooperate within the healing process. Her goal is to provide the optimum environment, internal and external, for the patient and co-workers of the helping professions. She knows and accepts that rivalry, antagonism, devaluation of individuals, and guarded communication minimize the effectiveness of restorative processes.

Complete nursing activity exacts the triumvirate activity of hands, head, and heart. It also includes consideration of the manner in which help is given, since the *way* in which it is extended affects patients.

At least three basic experiences occur to every ill person in some measure and are accentuated when that person is a patient in a hospital. These experiences are (1) feelings of isolation from the family, from the group society, or from the "old self"; (2) feelings of grief for the loss of health, for an impending loss of life, for the old life, or for the usually easy communion with well persons or the family; and (3) feelings of dependence, independence, and desires for interdependence and open communication with others. These feelings commonly arise through the acts of receiving, giving, and reciprocal giving and receiving and the need to maintain self-identity, to explore self-potentials, to enhance others, and to openly communicate.

DEPENDENCE AND ISOLATION

There is inherent in the state of illness the realization and reality of an individual's dependence and her aloneness. To encourage some independence, efforts are made to increase her feelings of self-worth and to support a degree of self-autonomy as her illness permits. This does not mean that all patients must be completely independent, even though they are transferred to self-care. Every ill individual, as every individual, is and must be dependent in varying degrees, times, and ways upon others. No ill person can be independent. She can be nurtured by learning that in illness she, as all other individuals, is *inter*dependent. In the illness situation this means that she and the helping-healing professions are interdependent, all relying on one another and working together for optimum healing. This implies reciprocal giving and receiving.

GRIEVING

If the future seems to indicate an unacceptable change in the self-image, in physical functioning, or in personal relationships, the individual may mourn or grieve for what has been lost to her. The incidence, magnitude, and duration of grief have been heretofore little recognized in the patient by nurses. Its manifestations are not dissimilar to a grief response to the death of a loved one. The stages of grief usually include a period of initial shock when the person may seem dazed or unable to comprehend what has happened or what is about to happen to her. The gynecologic patient may not "hear" her diagnosis, or she may not remember anything said after she hears it. After the emotional releases of crying or talking, the individual may be considered by others to be "taking it well" or facing up to her problems. If she indeed is grieving for the loss of her self-image or body image, her function of childbearing, or her ability to participate in marital relations, she may be almost completely preoccupied by her loss. The fact that she has a complete family and that more children had been vetoed long ago does not matter now. She has been denied something she once possessed, she is less than herself, she is not whole as she once was, and she mourns. She may be unable to express this except to wish she was again as she once was; since the present is dark and the future contains no remedy, she may talk and find comfort only in the past.

Feelings of depression, of guilt about a gynecologic disease, guilt of illness itself, or of pain may overlay the period of overwhelming loss and preoccupation. Anger may be directed toward herself (for delaying treatment), or her husband, or the doctor, or the nurse. Thus the mourning individual may be withdrawn from her visiting family or even angry with them. As with mourning a death, she may expect them to observe the mourning with her. Rather, they may be rejoicing over her recovery and approaching hospital discharge. She may fail to accept this as being as important as her unresolved loss and may perceive her family as not loving her, insensitive to her, or cruel to her suffering.

Time is required to grieve in order to restore the self-image and reevaluate relationships. If the marital relationship, for instance, has been good, the patient's ability to reestablish a sense of worth will not be difficult. Only when she has reestablished her world and herself in it will the mourning patient be able to turn away from self once more and to others.* However, in order to give once more she must have received support in her need from hospital personnel, family, and helping-healing professions.

GIVING AND RECEIVING

Giving and receiving are seen to be at the core of human interaction. To be able to give and to receive are as necessary in a state of health as in illness, dependence, independence, or grief.

The importance of these concepts is not of concern for the patient with illness alone but also for her family. They too experience isolation and loneliness, especially the loneliness of misunderstandings: their own new feelings and the patient's.

---

*Wright, M. Erik: The period of mourning in chronic illness. In Harrower, Molly, editor: Medical and psychological teamwork in the care of the chronically ill, Springfield, Ill., 1955, Charles C Thomas, Publisher, pp. 57-60.

They may mourn for the family that existed before the illness, for the individual before illness, or for the thwarted potential of the patient. They too hunger to give and receive in the midst of an environment that is little cognizant of their presence or the value of their presence. Nor is the student nurse or auxiliary personnel any different. In some measure their isolation in the hospital heirarchy is not dissimilar to the patient and her family. They need others, yet they need freedom to be themselves. They need open communication, yet they fear it, for it lays open their ignorance. They need to know what is happening and to partake in the activity. They need to receive in order to give. Certainly a nurse knows the act of giving, though not always why or how. How aware she is of the effect of her giving is often related to how she receives. That devaluation, shame, loss of face, or pride may be felt by patients as a result of acts of giving focuses attention on a facet of nursing often ignored. These concepts will be developed throughout future chapters.

•   •   •

The book has been divided into several sections. The basic objective has been to expose the many uniquenesses and commonalities of gynecologic patients that may influence the way help is extended to the individual, involving both the giver and the recipient. Throughout the book the three basic concepts of isolation, dependence, and mourning have been developed to expose their frequent combinations in the gynecologic patient.

In Chapter 2 the common symptoms of the gynecologic patient are identified: symptoms that impart meaning or significance to both patient and observer (either nurse or family) and therefore influence perception, communication, and how help is extended to the patient. In Chapters 3 and 4 are identified some of the changes inherent in a surgical patient that necessitate a changing perspective of the patient day by day and sometimes hour by hour. Giving to her and her family during these times will change accordingly. Dependence and independence in the adolescent, adult, and older adult patient produce varying effects on each individual nurse and provoke varying measures of giving. The influences inherent in gross age groups are explored in Chapters 5 to 7. Chapter 8 is devoted to the gynecologic patient who may be unable to give anything in return and seemingly affords few nursing satisfactions and few feelings of accomplishment: the cancer and/or research patient.

Sequential development of the original concepts and gynecologic symptomatology has been attempted throughout all chapters, adapting and developing it within new situations. Throughout, it has been our objective to help the nurse to begin to recognize her own feelings, sometimes of vulnerability, as she cares for and gives to another woman who fears or grieves for her femininity.

RECOMMENDED READINGS FOR STUDENTS

Lindbergh, Anne Morrow: Gift from the sea, New York, 1955, Pantheon Books, Inc., Chapter 3.

Westberg, Granger E.: Minister and doctor meet, New York, 1961, Harper & Row, Publishers, pp. 98-105.

Wright, M. Erik: The period of mourning in chronic illness. In Harrower, Molly, editor: Medical and psychological teamwork in the care of the chronically ill, Springfield, Ill., 1955, Charles C Thomas, Publisher, pp. 57-60.

RECOMMENDED READINGS FOR INSTRUCTORS

Cockerill, Eleanor: The interdependence of the professions in helping people, Social Casework **34:**371-378, 1953.

Neisser, Marianne: The two must face a third, Social Casework **39:**27-29, 1958.

Chapter 2

The patient's symptoms

Symptoms are guides or indicators to the helping professions that help is needed by the patient. Their intensity, sequence of occurrence, and duration are evaluated in order to make judgments and diagnoses and to prescribe therapy. Symptoms are also indicators to the patient and are interpreted by her, either accurately or inaccurately, rationally or irrationally. Because of this, the patient is unable to be completely objective in her reporting. Her communication, which may be verbal or nonverbal, is subjectively affected by the way she perceives her symptoms *and* by the person with whom she currently interacts. This means that symptoms are constantly being expressed or censored according to the way they "seem" to the observer and are expressed or censored to suit the hearer's ears or personality, whether that person is of one of the professions or not. Thus a subjectively experienced symptom automatically undergoes certain changes as the informant seeks to communicate.

The patient's past experience and/or cultural knowledge of a symptom, its present and future implications, and the listener can influence the ways the content will be shared. It may be complete, censored, accurate, or exaggerated. The information is further interpreted and censored in many ways by the listener, who may be the doctor or nurse. If either relates it to another, the content may be again censored. If their experience or cultural background has been dissimilar and if this is not recognized, the related symptom may be minimized or accentuated. The listener's perception and subjective opinion of the patient, the immediate circumstance in which the communication takes place, and the implied implications of the symptoms to the patient (or to the listener) will be powerful influences in an accurate or distorted interpretation of the communication. For example, if the patient is fearful of being misunderstood or of invoking impatience, the message may never be attempted, or it may be censored to achieve approval and understanding. If a nurse believes that a patient exaggerates her pain, the patient's verbal expressions or her nonverbal restlessness may be discounted. If a nurse is embarrassed by the thought of labial or vaginal pruritus, she may not seek to have the restlessness of a patient further interpreted. The patient's message may be ignored or repressed.

If symptoms are indeed guides and indicators to the helping-healing professions of help needed and its extent, then an understanding of symptoms and their meanings to both patients and nurses must be important. A foundation for this understanding forms the basis of this chapter, which includes the common gynecologic symptoms of bleeding, pruritus, and pain.

BLEEDING

Bleeding remains one of the most anxiety-laden symptoms. Bleeding is always subjectively experienced by the patient since it is a powerful stressor, and often it may be seen objectively by the patient and others. Observed bleeding produces anxiety or overt fear. Nonobserved bleeding, too, is anxiety producing, as demonstrated by the apprehensiveness of the patient who is hemorrhaging internally.

Bleeding may also be considered an extremely stress-laden symptom for the observer. Blood carries the universal connotation of being a life-giving and life-maintaining substance. Its loss therefore becomes life threatening. In the presence of bleeding there is a universal sense of emergency and an unmistakable drive to "do something." With successful control of bleeding, this feeling is completely absolved; the emergency is over. In the presence of uncontrolled and prolonged bleeding, anxiety is magnified. This shows itself in ineffectual haste, frenzy, controlled fury, random activity, helplessness, and/or dismay. The presence of bleeding is an ever-present and powerful stressor that involves *everyone* concerned.

Bleeding is a frequent gynecologic symptom. Its presence as the periodic bleeding of menstruation may elicit subjective apprehension and fear of uncontrolled bleeding in the young adolescent who is completely unprepared for the amount of blood involved. Student nurses recall:

> You think of what your mother tells you, "You're going to bleed a little bit each month," and you *think* you know what she means. It will be as if you prick your finger —six drops or something. Then, here it is, and you think you're hemorrhaging!

> My mother told me five or six months before, but actually I guess I didn't absorb it. When I started I was so disturbed; I thought I was bleeding to death.

While apprehension does not apparently persist in most women, it may be observed whenever periodicity becomes irregular, the usual flow increases, or the flow is accompanied by clotted blood.

The female nurse often feels personally threatened when there is abnormal and profuse bleeding and large clots. Nurse and patient are involved in a common vulnerability. How objective then is the nurse's judgment or evaluation of the amount of the patient's bleeding? What is her concept of the normal bleeding amount? Is it based on the patient's past history of bleeding? Is it based on the "usual textbook amount"? Is it based on her own personal experience? Some European cultures equate a heavy flow with fertility. Is a student nurse from such a cultural background less aware of the anxiety of a patient who experiences an unusually profuse flow? How accurately will she evaluate the extent of the bleeding; that is, if a heavy flow is "good," will she subjectively tend to minimize an abnormally heavy amount?

Since evaluation of gynecologic bleeding is usually a subjective measurement, any subjective factors influencing the perception of the nurse are pertinent. They become individual foci for self-knowledge and for awareness and knowledge of others by student, staff, supervisor, and instructor.

Systemic effects of bleeding

The systemic responses to the loss of blood involve the interactions of the sympathetic-parasympathetic nervous systems, respiratory system, endocrine system, renal mechanisms, and the circulatory system itself. The immediate response to injury and bleeding is an increase of epinephrine and norepinephrine. They produce the first compensatory mechanisms for a diminishing blood volume: a constriction of peripheral vessels (those not supplying blood to vital areas which are therefore expendable as a conservation measure), an increased vascular resistance, and an increased cardiac stroke volume.

These functions are seen in the patient as pallor, a small rise in diastolic blood pressure, and an increased pulse rate. If bleeding is severe, increased norepinephrine will clinically produce skin moistness (not very conservative), and the patient may feel cold due to diminished peripheral circulation and body heat loss. A diminishing blood volume will be reflected in a weak pulse in addition to the accentuated rate. If all compensatory mechanisms fail, the systolic blood pressure will drop. Diminishing blood volume directly affects the oxygenation of cells; therefore, the respiratory center is stimulated and an increased respiratory rate ensues.

Diminished blood volume and renal vasoconstriction in response to the bleeding drastically reduces the glomerular filtration pressure, and water conservation is accomplished. The antidiuretic hormone may also function here. Increased aldosterone influences the increased resorption of sodium and water and the increased excretion of potassium. The accompanying change in the fluid volume and electrolytes results in the patient's thirst.

Evaluation of vital signs is necessary to determine the clinical progress of the patient who is bleeding. The initial reaction of epinephrine and norepinephrine on an increased pulse rate and an increased diastolic pressure may be a good indication of the extent of the initial bleeding. Factors of fear and excitement, some of which may be absorbed by the patient from the personnel, may muddle the picture. Since continued bleeding and a decreased blood volume will influence the cardiac stroke volume (Starling's law), the pulse rate becomes even more rapid. The systolic blood pressure may and probably will remain stable. Reduced blood volume and an increased heart rate increase the respiratory rate. Thus the *first signs* of new bleeding may be increased pulse, increased respirations, and increasing diastolic pressure. The slowly rising diastolic pressure indicates increasing peripheral resistance, an *early* response to a diminishing blood volume. By the time the systolic pressure falls, all other compensatory mechanisms have failed and shock is present.

Observations and evaluation of the total interrelationship of vital signs are necessary, if "*taking* vital signs" is to be of more significance than just that. Inherent in the delegation of observing vital signs to the nurse is the valid assumption that she is capable of interpreting their significance within the clinical situation. In the absence of her ability to make these judgments, vital signs "taken" by a nurse become only a collection of useless data and mounting "things to do."

Hemostatic process

Prevention and control of bleeding are dependent on a complex interaction of many factors, without which loss of blood would be possible with every minor bump or pressure, and bleeding, once it had begun, would continue unabated. The specific importance of the various processes involved in hemostatic control seems to be in direct relation to the size of the vessel involved, the amount of the vascularization of the area, and therefore, the blood flow within that part. In a small vessel the immediate constriction of the vessel and the accumulation, agglutination, and disintegration of platelets at the site may be enough to afford hemostasis. However, when a large vessel (artery or vein) is affected, control of bleeding is dependent on the efficiency of the entire hemostatic mechanism.

As vital to survival as hemostasis may be, regulatory factors that control the extent and duration of the blood coagulability are equally vital. Therefore, the total mechanism is a delicate balance. Continued fibrin formation or continued presence of a formed clot would result in multiple thrombic formations or total vessel occlusion. The mechanisms that control this dangerous possibility are the anticoagulants and the fibrinolytic system. This system is involved in the non-clotting quality of menstrual blood.

Uterine bleeding

The majority of gynecologic diseases associated with abnormal uterine bleeding can be diagnosed or at least suggested by the patient's history alone. Prolonged profuse menses suggests fibroids or glandular dysfunction; postmenopausal bleeding means carcinoma of the endometrium or cervix until proved otherwise; postcoital and intermenstrual spotting signals carcinoma of the cervix. Bleeding in the child-bearing years suggests a complication of pregnancy. (Fig. 1.) The history of bruising, bleeding from the gums when brushing the teeth, and undue bleeding after a surgical procedure suggest systemic causes of the bleeding such as thrombocytopenic purpura or leukemia.

The patient operated upon may often be anguished and worried at the onset

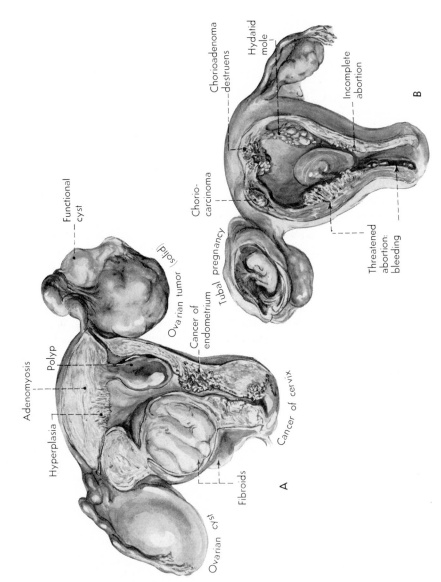

Fig. 1. Causes of abnormal uterine bleeding. **A,** Gynecologic bleeding. **B,** Complications of pregnancy associated with bleeding. If there are no pathologic, hematologic, or endocrinologic causes for the abnormal bleeding, the bleeding is classified as dysfunctional.

of an irregular period of uterine bleeding soon after her operation. Whether this operation did or did not involve a gynecologic procedure, she may not understand why she bleeds and may fear further physical problems.

In an individual in optimum health a periodic 23- to 34-day cycle of menstrual bleeding occurs. This blood is unclotted and usually amounts to about 25 to 50 ml.

Nursing implications

The effect the nurse and doctor have upon the patient and family cannot be underestimated as they work to control bleeding or as they examine the patient. As they talk to the patient and family or as they express themselves by gesture or facial expression, the patient may receive trust and assurance or fear and uncertainty of impending tragedy. In like manner, frequent observation of vital signs may either reassure the patient or create mounting terror that she is bleeding to death or that her bleeding is not medically controllable. What is communicated through the voice, body movements, and hands of the nurse and other individuals in contact with the patient to some extent will determine her response.

Another consideration for nursing activity in the presence of bleeding is an awareness of the effect of the physical environment on the patient. The bleeding patient may feel very isolated and frightened. She may be more frightened in a private room, yet she may be jumpy and anxious in the presence of roommates or visitors. Sensitive nurses develop skill in matching roommates who will have a synergistic action with one another. This is an anticipatory maneuver enacted *before* it is necessary to move the patient because of detrimental environmental effects. The location of the room of a bleeding patient may also be an important factor. The patient's anxiety will usually be reduced if she feels that her room or her bed placement within the room is visible and available to the hub of activity, that is, the nursing station or at least the hallway nearby. It is important that staff members frequently pause at the door or look in as they pass. Such activity, rather than overstimulating or denying the patient rest, administers confidence to the patient that she is being watched closely and that she is safe. She can therefore *allow* herself to rest and to go to sleep. The anticipation and accomplishment of these factors are pertinent nursing measures.

The patient may be embarrassed in a room with others or in the presence of visitors because of frequent bed soiling or the distinct odor of blood. Continued anxiety from this cause, along with fear of the bleeding itself, is detrimental to the patient. Their alleviation is within the area of control of a sensitive and competent nurse. The role of the nurse is to act as a buffer between these forces and the patient in order to conserve the patient's strength, which is needed to cope with her stress situation.

PRURITUS

The itching patient is most uncomfortable; once the itch cycle takes over, her anguish may become almost a frenzy. She also creates "itchy" feelings in the observer. Itching patients are not usually "good" patients (1) because they *do* make the observer uncomfortable, (2) because all attempts to alleviate itching may be ineffectual, and (3) because they do not stop scratching. Thus medical personnel often avoid the itching patient or make personal contacts short and only when necessary. This only further accentuates the patient's anxiety, resentment, and embarrassment for her need to scratch and accentuates her itching and further rejection.

Itch is therefore seen to be composed of two aspects: it may have an initial physical stimulus component or *input* in addition to a psychologic component to interpret the sensation as an itch and instigate action. The latter component is the *output* or *processing* component. (As may be appreciated, physical itch may arise as an emotional or intellectual stimulus.)

Pruritus in the gynecologic patient arises locally in the area of the vulva and vagina as a result of infections. These may be caused by the organisms of yeast *(Candida albicans), Trichomonas vaginalis,* or *Pseudomonas vaginalis.* Vulvar pruritus may develop when late postmenopausal tissue changes occur, with malignant and premalignant changes, or with systemic diseases.

Infection and gynecologic itching are closely associated in the patient's mind. Because infection of gynecologic origin initially contains a "shame" connotation, some patients delay seeking help with this symptom until they can no longer bear the discomfort.

Local pruritus in other than gynecologic areas may be experienced by the gynecologic patient who has had x-ray therapy. This may remain localized to the area of therapy, or the itching sensation and urge to scratch may involve other areas of the body in addition.

Generalized pruritus may also be experienced by the gynecologic patient who has an allergic response to antibiotics or administered blood.

Input component

The origin of somatic itch is dependent on (1) the initial stimulus, (2) the activity of mediators, (3) the stimulation of small terminal endings of the nerve fibers, and (4) the transmission of the impulse to the cortex for an identification of "itch."

The primary stimulus arises at the terminal endings of nerve C fibers in *intact* epidermis or mucous membrane. It is a result of (1) the direct tactile stimulation of the nerve endings by very light stroking or minimal touch, as may be remembered by the "feel" of gnats flying against the sensitive nerve endings of the face, or (2) tissue injury with the liberation of tissue enzymes. Whether such agents directly excite the nerve endings or whether they alter the nerve ending sensitivity is still being investigated.

Sensory nerve fibers are classified according to their size. Small fibers (C fibers) have slow conduction; large fibers (A fibers) have rapid conduction. Impulses interpreted as "itch" by the cerebral cortex are carried in the C fibers. The threshold for C fibers is a hundred times greater than A fibers. There are four times as many C fibers as A fibers.

Output or processing component

Itch, like pain, is not a sensory perception. It is comprehended by the cortex. Thus the response to itch is influenced by many factors.

The response to itch or itching may be modified by the significance of the "feeling" of itching to the individual, the presence of fatigue or coexistent pain, the amount of attention directed to it, and the degree of cultural and sociologic acceptance of the act itself.

New itching or a continuation of itching to a fatigued and exasperated patient will be accentuated through greater cerebral feedback, with very little if any added peripheral stimulus.

Whether the patient scratches or not is dependent on her cultural environment and its disciplinary implications. Thus an old English proverb says, " 'Tis better than riches to scratch when it itches," but the seventeenth century gentlewoman tapped rather than scratched. There are strict taboos of scratching certain body areas.

The ability and the will to itch are finally determined by the cerebral cortex. The output or processing center (cortex) is capable of a summation and accentuation of the sensation itself, with little if any additional peripheral stimulus. This may be appreciated by remembering the ease with which a previously itch-free individual may begin to "feel" itchy only through observation of excessive and prolonged scratching or the appearance of itchy-looking skin. It also means that *itching in one area may be experienced and expressed as generalized itching.* Cortical arousal may also arise through the emotions of anger and fear, which create changes in epidermal circulation and perhaps create cellular production of proteases or polypeptides, physical stimuli for pruritus.

Regardless of the kind of itch stimulus or its source, any itch is action directed toward mediation of the causal irritant or the itch itself. The motor response for relief of the irritant may be scratching with the nails, rubbing one extremity against another, the use of any object to reach the area, pinching, slapping, and actual mutilation and destruction of tissue. After excessive scratching, itch cannot be elicited for 15 to 20 minutes since scratching or rubbing damages superficial C fiber nerve endings of the epidermis or mucous membrane and they cannot be stimulated until they grow again. With their destruction, A fibers are stimulated and bright burning pain or sharp pain ensues.

Nursing implications

After removal of the causal agent of pruritus, all medical treatment and nursing extended to the patient with symptoms of itching are directed toward minimizing further "insult to injury" from the scratching action, reducing further itching and reducing anxiety and physical injury. Therapy and nursing may be arbitrarily divided into those measures that seek to control or inhibit pruritus by (1) decreasing the inflow of stimuli, (2) changing the output or processing component by modifying the interpretation of the impulse, and (3) providing restorative measures for denuded or injured tissue areas with protection from secondary infection.

Decreasing inflow of stimuli. Local anesthetic ointments or injectable agents may be used for the intractable itching of the gynecologic patient. They desensitize the C fibers at the genesis of the input component.

Pressure stimulates the large myelinated A fibers which oppress the C fibers. Therefore, firm pressure over or proximal to the pruritic area (pubis) will beneficially reduce itching. This may be explained to the patient so that she will minimize the destructive means to which most patients eventually resort for relief. Conversely, all light touch stimulates the C fibers. Filmy clothing as well as rough clothing seams may provide stimuli. Clothing should be scrutinized by the nurse, family, and patient, with a critical view toward its effect on the itching cycle. The patient's contact with sheets at night may also enhance itching. A cradle may be necessary to keep the top sheet from touching the shins or shoulders. Firm touch should be used when giving injections, awakening the sleeping patient, supporting her out of bed or walking, and giving back rubs with an *emollient*. Feathery and tantalizing tactile stimuli arouse new waves of itching.

All nervous tissue is more excitable with heat; C fibers are more sensitive as heat increases capillary dilatation of epidermis or mucous membrane. Thus cold applications for intermittent periods of 30 minutes will abolish itching. Continuous and sporadic applications of local cold, however, stimulate secondary vasodilatation, with a resumption of itching.

Similarly, water used by the patient for bathing should be cool. Cool tub baths in a comfortably warmed room are to be preferred to showers, which produce multiple peripheral stimuli by the jets of water and reactivate itching. Water dripping off a washcloth onto the skin or running down the back or arms may provide new stimuli. Patients should wash with firm strokes to minimize fine tactile stimuli, and they should dry with firm blotting pressure, using a linen towel rather than the harsh stimulation of a turkish towel. Sudden temperature changes during bathing are to be avoided, since the activity of shivering raises the skin temperature and new itching can resume.

Many of the aforementioned precautions for resumption of itching seem very unrelated when applied to the gynecologic patient. However, C fiber stimuli on any part of the body may diffuse to a temporarily latent site by means of the spreading input component, or because the cortex interprets one itch the same as another. Soon the patient has a resumption of the original pruritus. She may in addition "itch" all over.

Modifying interpretation. Fatigue, anxiety, embarrassment, resentment, excitement, and therefore stress increase the cortical response to incoming stimuli, with an accelerated summation feedback to the cortex. Since all these factors are present in most patients with pruritus, optimum environment and interpersonal relationships are especially important. For instance, protection of the patient from nap disturbances during the day will permit her the rest she often is unable to obtain at night. The many soothing rituals of preparing the individual for sleep are important as well as a relaxed and nonstimulating (as opposed to a harried or noisy) environment. In contrast to the patient in pain, the itching patient seldom seems to like isolation and benefits from mutual interpersonal relationships. She is often an "unpopular patient" and ashamed, often unable to speak of her discomfort and misery, and often acutely feels the discomfort and embarrassment of the staff in contact with her.

Mandatory rules and punitive "don't's" rouse new waves of "itch" followed by scratching. It is as unrealistic to say, "don't scratch" as it is to say "don't get excited" to a hypertensive patient or "don't forget" to a hypothyroid patient.

Tranquilizers are frequently used to reduce the anxiety attendant with all itching. They reduce the significance of the itching to the patient; she does not worry about itching and so itches less.

In the presence of pain, itching is blocked. At night, as the distractions of the day fall away and an administered analgesic becomes effective, the pain-free, tired patient may begin to itch more severely than she ever did during daytime hours. At least four factors may accelerate the symptom: increased attention to the symptom, fatigue, freedom from pain, and the warmth of the bedding. Sometimes cold dry applications are the only means of relief for the patient at night.

Providing restorative measures for denuded tissue areas. Restorative measures for denuded tissue areas involve cleanliness of the area from contaminating discharges and wastes from other orifices and medications by local application or systemic administration. Secondary infection in denuded skin surfaces without natural defenses is to be avoided.

It is difficult to care for an individual when the magnitude of the disease and its effect on the feelings of the patient are incomprehensible to the nurse or doctor. It is also difficult to care for an individual when the personnel begin to share the patient's symptom. Instead of running from them, perhaps all such patients afford us unlimited possibilities to explore the unknown regions of empathic relationships.

PAIN

Of all symptoms, pain seems to present the greatest barrier to effective and accurate communication between the patient and the nonpatient. This has important implications for members of the healing professions for whom pain is at once a common patient symptom and still one that is little understood and that cannot be experienced by them in its present state.

Pain presents the members of the healing professions with ever-present dilemmas: they are uncomfortable if pain is not acknowledged by the patient or if pain is absent when its presence is expected; they want to administer medications to alleviate suffering, yet they may be uncertain and/or reluctant to do so under such circumstances.

The symptoms of pain *always* demand the formulation of a judgment concerning that pain by the doctor and the nurse. *Each* is required to evaluate the following: the character of the patient's pain, its locale, and the direction of its radiation; the intensity of the pain and its duration; and its manner of onset and the aggravating factors. They also evaluate the diagnostic implications of the pain, comparing it with similar clinical experiences and comparing it with the past pain experiences of the patient; the presence of coexisting and contributing influences on the pain, such as anxiety or fatigue, and the effect of a therapeutic treatment or of personnel on the pain expression; the indications for various nursing measures; and the kind of analgesic indicated for the patient's pain at this particular time and its effect on the future activity of the patient, such as ambulation, postoperative coughing, eating, or sleeping. They evaluate the frequency of the medication to be given the patient with this pain and whether the pain characteristics should be further observed rather than masked by an analgesic.

> We do not approach any problem with a wholly naive or virgin mind; we approach it with certain acquired habitual modes of understanding, with a certain store of previously evolved meanings or at least of experiences from which meanings may be educed. . . . No hard and fast rules decide whether a meaning suggested is the right and proper meaning to follow up. The individual's own good (or bad) judgment is the guide. There is no label on any given idea or principle which says automatically, "Use me in this situation"—as the magic cakes of Alice in Wonderland were inscribed, "Eat me." The thinker has to decide, to choose; and there is always a risk, so that the prudent thinker selects warily. . . . If one is not able to estimate wisely what is relevant to the interpretation of a given perplexing or doubtful issue, it avails little that arduous learning has built up a large stock of concepts. For learning is not wisdom; information does not guarantee good judgment. Memory may provide an antiseptic refrigerator in which to store a stock of meanings for future use, but judgment selects and adopts the one to be used. . . .*

In order to begin to evaluate all factors and to formulate a judgment about the patient's pain and its alleviation, the healing professions must rely on the *ability* of the patient to describe her pain and her *willingness* to do so.

Willingness of the patient to communicate pain

Before anyone is able to communicate with another, she must in some manner quickly identify with that other person. Thus a patient "sizes up" a nurse; she tries "to tune her in to her own wavelength" in an effort to determine how best to communicate with this particular nurse. The patient attempts to ascertain (1) if the nurse is interested in her: will she *hear* her message? (2) if she is understanding: will she sympathetically *accept* and correctly *interpret* her message? and (3) if she is knowledgeable: will she appropriately fulfill the request of her message?

To achieve this thumbnail impression of another person the patient may give

---

*Dewey, John: How we think, Boston, 1910, D. C. Heath & Co., pp. 106-107.

honor to the saying "Actions speak louder than words" and look first to body actions and gestures as more accurate indicators of purpose and meaning. Through facial clues she may believe she sees kindness, interest, sadness, distraction, impatience, annoyance, or displeasure. Through the nurse's manner of approaching the bedside, the patient may decide the nurse's willingness to come, her concern, or her reluctance, or she may decide, "She's just answering another light." The patient may evaluate the distance the nurse stands from the bedside as aloofness, uneasiness, ready incorporation into the situation, or assuredness; she may evaluate the body and hand movements of the nurse as competent, deft, tender, willing, unsure, fearful, hesitant, angry, or clumsy. She may place value on her observance that a nurse looks at her first and the gadgetry second or that a nurse may be occupied with the mechanics *and* with her at the same time. Modulation of voice, articulation, speech mannerisms, and expressive content give the patient further clues that she integrates into her whole picture of the nurse with whom she must now communicate her pain.

If she has decided (correctly or incorrectly) that the nurse is kind, but hurried and tired, she may devalue her pain or play it down—"I don't want to cause any more trouble for her." A student nurse commented, "Lots of patients just won't complain when they're having pain. You have to ask or observe them. If I say, 'Shall I get you something for pain now?' they'll say, 'Yes'; but they would have lain there all morning rather than ring for you because they'll say, 'Well, I thought you were so busy.' "

If she has decided that the nurse is harried, apprehensive, aloof, or aggravated, she may also devalue her pain, for she may not feel it worth the effort to defend her message. However, when the patient does feel it necessary to communicate her pain to this same nurse, she may *over*emphasize it. In other words, the patient may turn up the volume and repeat her message like an SOS signal, attempting to get the message through even the poor reception of this nurse.

If the patient has decided that the nurse is kind, but inexperienced and apprehensive, the patient may try to control the uncertain or unsafe interpretation of her message by direct request or demand what she needs (a medication or a nursing measure) without telling about the pain at all; or to this nurse this patient may freely confide her fear of the pain or her explanation for the reasons for her pain and illness. The patient may feel such expressions might bring censor or derision from a more experienced nurse.

If the patient has decided that the nurse is understanding, deft, and unhurried, she may feel free to cry; she may feel confident to verbally describe her pain as adequately as she can express it, supplemented with gestures or other cues; or she may feel so relieved and compliant that she may completely abdicate making any further evaluations and decisions and agree to any and all of the nurse's interpretations and suggestions. "Just do anything, nurse. I know I'm in good hands now."

Each patient's *mode* and *content* of expression are influenced by each nurse with whom the patient communicates. Patients try to speak the language they believe the listener will understand and what they want to hear. If they think the listener places higher significance on communication that is objectively related, the patient will strive to communicate her pain in this manner, even though it may grossly distort what she wants to say. Patients try to be "good patients" according to their own standard of "good" and according to the interpreted expectations of them by hospital personnel, collectively and individually. Patients fear the loss of goodwill of the hospital personnel and possible abandonment and/or retaliations if it does occur.* The content and language used to describe pain are *censored* in a certain way by the patient as she communicates with each person about that pain. This emphasizes the necessity for *frequent* nurse-patient interactions, not only limited to medication-dispensing times.

Ability of the patient to communicate pain

The patient communicates pain verbally and nonverbally.

Verbal communication of pain. Verbal language is especially inadequate in those emotionally experienced situations that cannot be experienced or participated in by others. Pain is an emotionally experienced situation. It is known only by the sufferer.

A patient verbally communicates her introspective thoughts and feelings about pain in different frames of reference. As she purposely strives for a common language to express her unique feelings of pain, she uses adjectives, analogies, similes, and experiences known to most people.

Patient may give pain a quality. The patient uses the nouns and adjectives of crick, stitch, twinge, sharp, burning, stinging, aching, piercing, biting, grinding, pinching, shooting, throbbing, or gnawing to describe pain. Some of these words refer to an action such as piercing and shooting, which is then imagined as similar to the pain situation. Some of the words seem to preclude previous experience of similar pain in order to be able to use the word with accuracy or to comprehend its meaning. That is, a *stinging* pain or an *aching* pain has meaning only to someone who has had a sting or an ache before, in contrast to a darting pain, which could be imagined as one that is elusive and fleeting. Perhaps this is the basis for the poverty of the child's language of pain and also that of some adults inexperienced with pain, who can only say, "It hurts," "I have pain," or "I'm in misery." Nurses and doctors who try to help the patient describe her pain often suggest words of description to them. There is no reason to believe that such descriptive words are understood or interpreted *in the same way* by the patient, especially by the patient unaccustomed to pain or by one who experiences visceral pain for the first time.

In a study of experimental pain in which increasingly different intensities of pain stimuli were given the subjects, one subject reported "sharp" to the minimal

---

*Visotsky, Harold M., Hamburg, David A., Goss, Mary E., and Lebovits, Binyamin Z.: Coping behavior under extreme stress, Archives of General Psychiatry **5:**431, 1961.

stimuli and "soreness like an open cut" to the maximal pain stimuli.* In a clinical setting it would have been important for the nurse to be able to interpret the language of this "patient." The report of "sharpness" and "soreness" not only indicated a *quality* of pain present but also (in this case) indicated a change in *intensity* or *severity*. Unless constant reinterpretation and verification of the communication persisted between the nurse and the patient, the nurse may have been ignorant of the intended meaning of increasing pain.

Patient tries to give pain a quantity, an intensity. In order to quantify pain a patient is required to compare her pain. If she says, "My pain is severe or hard," she is saying that, compared with some remembered past pain, *this one* is severe. She describes her pain as an *absolute* measure. Yet patients have difficulty remembering past pain. "Pain itself passes and is quickly forgotten: we cannot recall the sensation. . . . Suffering passes, but the fact of having suffered never passes. A man acquainted with the terror of pain is irrevocably changed. . . . What is the reason for the change in his behaviour, the modification in his judgment, his new attitude to things, to people, to himself?"† In addition, we are unable to know the patient's experience and her comparative measure of pain. All types of pain are not the same even to the same individual. The significance attached to a specific pain increases or decreases its experienced intensity. Compared to the anxiety and fear prior to operation, the surgical patient may regard her postoperative pain as bearable, expected, or even minor, for now she knows she will be all right. The older patient with life experiences of pain and the surgical patient are not necessarily saying that their pain at this time is insignificant and can be ignored, but rather that their pain experiences in life have been so great that the present pain pales in significance. A man lost in the mountains and deprived of food for a week considers a later imposed fast of two days in the hospital insignificant in comparison, although his two-day hunger is real.

A patient may also attempt to quantify pain by comparing her present pain with the "remembered" original. Thus she may decide, "I have less pain," a *relative* measure. A nurse may interpret this as pain relief. Lasagna raises an interesting question: What is pain relief? Is it *any* degree of relief, complete relief, or at least 50% relief? His study indicated that patients considered relief from severe pain to moderate pain most important to them. This is called "patient gratitude" for relief of pain from one level to another. Relief was considered least important from slight pain to the absence of pain. Most important for the nurse is the reported finding that patients placed a lesser value on relief of very severe pain to severe pain.‡ If patients indeed place less importance in a *little* pain relief when

---

*Smith, Robert: The vocabulary of pain. In Keele, C. A., editor: The assessment of pain in man and animals, London, 1962, E. & S. Livingstone, Ltd., p. 38.

†Buytendijk, F. J. J.: Pain, its modes and functions, Chicago, 1962, University of Chicago Press, p. 28. (Translated by Eda O'Shiel.)

‡Lasagna, Louis: The clinical measurement of pain, Annals of the New York Academy of Sciences **86:**28-37, 1960.

they have maximum pain, do they cease to communicate with us during this time? If so, is their minimal verbal communication or its absence accepted as a "moderately comfortable" patient or even as a pain-free, uncomplaining patient?

Nurses may erroneously quantify pain when they judge the sleeping patient as the pain-free patient. She may be an anxiety-free patient or a pain-exhausted patient who sleeps, but nontheless has pain.

Patient may try to place pain in a spatial relationship of time and place. The patient may locate pain precisely by naming the offending organ or region: "pain in my back," "mittleschmerz," etc. Gestures verify these locations and help the patient and the observer understand exactly where. Gynecologic pain is often difficult for the patient to locate and delineate. She may identify pain in seemingly unrelated structures such as back, hips, legs, and the region of the umbilicus. She may indicate diffusion of her pain, "pain all over," by using hand gestures for definitive location. Thus the patient whose hands may be restrained or immobilized by an intravenous infusion and lateral positioning feels seriously handicapped in communicating her pain. This is particularly true of the patient striving to communicate "deep" pain or visceral pain.

A patient may describe time frequencies of pain as steady, comes and goes, or gone for "awhile." Doctors and nurses superimpose upon her vocabulary such words as intermittent, constant, and acute and the time-limiting boundaries of pain duration in minutes or hours. But to the patient,

> Pain has an element of Blank;
> It cannot recollect
> When it began—or if there were
> A time when it was not.*

Nonverbal communication of pain. Americans are inclined to ignore nonverbal communication, giving most emphasis to verbal content. However, nonverbal language or the communication rendered by gestures, facial expression, and body action becomes the priority language in times of physical or emotional crises and in those situations in which words are inadequate or unavailable.

The physical cues of pain are those resulting from the autonomic nervous system response to pain. These are increased pulse rate, paleness, increased respirations, perspiration, and dilated pupils. Facial changes of the set jaw, furrowed brow, or grimace are well recognized. Body rigidity, guarding of a part, retraction of the leg to minimize abdominal pain, random and purposeless movements, complete motionlessness, or the hidden clenched hand are frequently overlooked nonverbal expressions of pain.

As these actions, gestures, or cues are identified, an evaluation must be made by the observer regarding the patient's meaning or intent, and a comparison must be made with what the patient says verbally. Nonverbal cues usually substantiate

---

*Dickinson, Emily: In Johnson, Thomas H., editor: The complete poems of Emily Dickinson, Boston: 1960, Little, Brown & Co., p. 323.

or intensify the verbal expression. Accurate interpretation of a patient's communication includes consideration of *both* verbal and nonverbal content.

When there is discrepancy between verbal expression and nonverbal language, such as the verbal denial of pain by the patient accompanied by nonverbal cues of pain, the nurse may continue to try to interpret these two discrepancies and to seek further clues or to verify one or the other pain language. A student nurse comments, "When I say to patients, 'Do you have pain?' and they say, 'No,' then I accept it. But if they say, 'No, it's okay,' I think perhaps there's something else there. It's the *way* they say it." The voice inflection becomes the discordant communication signal in this example, and the nurse looks for further cues or other interviewing techniques to reconcile the patient's verbal and nonverbal languages.

In the presence of a discrepancy between verbal and nonverbal expression, a nurse may accept the one she believes the more "reliable" as the valid patient communication and may ignore the other conflicting or incongruent one. In the presence of strong emotional cues, the trembling mouth or the clenched hands, pain intensity is inferred, and the nonverbal expression gains precedence over its verbal content. As emotion increases, nonverbal language becomes completely dominant, and the nurse minimizes all verbal content. Crying is a universal emergency language. "In daily life, human beings are rarely able to do more than to hint at what they desire to express, inasmuch as the very nature of their needs often forces them to exchange messages without delay in time. Thus it is left to the receiver to fill in unexpressed details."*

The patient's experience of pain

Pain is not only difficult for the patient to explain but has become increasingly complex for the investigator and clinician to interpret. Experimental work has revealed the interplay of many factors in the pain experience. Many of these are important for an improved understanding of the patient in pain, the environment in which pain exists, and applied methods of pain alleviation.

Recent investigations by Beecher raise serious question that the pain experience is the same in animal and man and question that experimentally produced pain is the same as clinically experienced pain. The pain experience, like itch, is believed to be comprised of two components: (1) the *input component* or the instigation of nervous tissue stimulation by means of a noxious stimuli and (2) the *output* or *processing component* which interprets and censors the ensuing activity known as the pain expression or reaction.†

Input component. The anatomic pathways of the pain impulse travel from receptor endings to the reticular formation and cerebral cortex. As the nerve im-

---

*Ruesch, Jurgen, and Kees, Weldon: Non-verbal communication: Notes on the visual perception of human relations, Berkeley, 1964, University of California Press, p. 8.

†An extensive bibliography of these studies and a discussion of their significance may be obtained in Beecher, Henry K.: Measurement of subjective responses, New York, 1959, Oxford University Press.

pulses are interpreted and processed by the cerebrum, they become the recognized sensation of pain.

Pelvic pain may originate through pelvic muscle, fascia, and cutaneous innervation (lumbosacral plexus or sacral plexus) or through visceral innervation via the pathways of the sacral autonomic (parasympathetic) and the thoracolumbar autonomic (sympathetic) nervous systems.

Cutaneous and muscle innervation involves nerve fibers called A fibers. Pain arising from such areas is usually described by the patient as burning, stinging, sharp, or cutting. This pain can usually be located with some accuracy by the patient. The labia, vagina, and abdominal wall would originate pain of this character.

Visceral innervation involves nerve fibers called C fibers. These are slow conductors of the pain impulse, few in number compared to A fibers, and they are unmyelinated. Often pain originating in these fibers is referred pain. Thus pain arising in the uterus, ovary, tubes, bladder, and rectum may be experienced at the direct site of origin, but it also may be referred to other areas following neurodermatome segments. This means that the patient's identification of the focus of her pain may not always be the direct source but may be its referred site. The physical stimuli of vasoconstriction or smooth muscle distention in the presence of intact C fibers initiates a pain impulse. It is important to recognize that temperature, touch, or cutting are not thought to be pain stimuli to these nerve fibers. Thus a tenaculum may be used to grasp the cervix and a biopsy taken without anesthesia. Similarly, cauterization of the cervix is not experienced by the patient as burning or bright pain. If it is experienced at all as pain, it is described as an aching or deep, dull pain, and the location of this pain is usually experienced in the low back. This is *referred pain*. The pain of dysmenorrhea may be experienced as direct pain; that is, its location may be somewhat accurately described, or it too may be referred pain involving not only the pelvic area but also the low back, thighs, and legs.

Pelvic pain, therefore is often confused or distorted in its interpretation by the patient because of the way she experiences the pain. It is more difficult for her to describe quality, site, and severity of pain as it arises in the pelvis than other sources of pain. While pelvic pain may indicate a gynecologic problem, it also may be the symptom of orthopedic, genitourinary, or gastrointestinal tract disorders. Conversely, pain that seems to be an orthopedic symptom (back or knee pains), a genitourinary symptom (dysuria), or a gastrointestinal tract symptom (pain aggravated by defecation) may in reality be important gynecologic symptoms. Delay in seeking gynecologic help may often be due to these misinterpretations of her pain by the patient.

Output or processing component. This essential component in the pain experience determines the individual response or reaction to the sensation of pain. It is the influence exerted on the expression of the pain in the cerebral cortex by such factors as cultural or family expectations of a person in pain, her life experiences, her pain experiences, the physical, philosophic, or religious meaning of pain to her, or the meaning of the injury or disease itself that engendered the pain. This means that the pain threshold does not involve the receptor ending. Rather, the pain threshold or the reaction to pain varies from individual to individual and varies within a single individual, depending on how the pain sensation is conceptualized in the cerebral cortex. The processing component of pain seems to explain those individuals with a congenital insensitivity to pain, the use of hypnosis in the alleviation of pain, and the surgical procedure of leukotomy, which does not eliminate the sensation of pain but changes the importance of the pain to the patient and, therefore, the patient's response to the pain.

Significance of the wound. Studies of wounded soldiers in battle have shown a distortion between their reaction to pain and the seriousness of their wound. The extensiveness of the wounds should have precipitated great suffering; the processing component or the psychic reaction to the pain sensation minimized its expression in the presence of the greater emotion of safe removal from the battlefield.* In like manner, the gynecologic patient responds to pain according to the significance she accords her surgical wound. If it means to her the symbol of great loss, an uncertain future, and disrupted relationships, the significance of the wound is great, and the pain experience may be intense. Other strong emotions arising during the postoperative period could alter or block her response to pain if they can change the importance of the injury to the patient.

Significance of the pain. The relationship of pain and the significance of the pain itself may be seen in the reactions to pain by different nationality groups. Those who focus concern on the meaning of pain and its threat to health and security actively react to pain.† Those who anticipate pain react to pain. It is believed that analgesics act by reducing the anticipation of pain, thereby changing the behavior to pain. Morphine has been found effective only when given in the presence of the *anxiety* that it relieves. The pain *reaction* of the patient is then changed. Anticipation of pain in childbirth and menstruation is associated with increased pain reaction and often with long periods of dysmenorrhea. It is observed that dysmenorrhea in the nulliparous woman is sometimes *not* experienced in that woman after childbirth. Is this a changed pain reaction after the greater pain experiences of labor that devalue the periodic pain of menstruation?

To the cancer patient the presence of pain is equated with the persistence of the disease entity. Anxieties of uncertainty, of communication isolation from those who could help her, or of physical isolation from her loved ones can accentuate the pain experience. This increased pain experience may then engender greater

---

*Beecher, Henry K.: Relationship of the significance of the wound to the pain experienced, Journal of the American Medical Association **161:**1609-1613, 1956. Also in Beecher, Henry K.: Measurement of subjective responses, New York, 1959, Oxford University Press, pp. 164-165.

†Zborowski, Mark: Cultural components in responses to pain, Journal of Social Issues **8**(4):16-30, 1952. Also in Jaco, E. Gartly, editor: Patients, physicians and illness, New York, 1958, Free Press of Glencoe, Inc., pp. 256-268.

feelings about the meaning of the pain severity. Increased anxieties result, followed by increased pain. "Cancer pain is often most unbearable because hope, understanding, and personal interest have been withheld, consciously or unconsciously, from the patient by his physician or nursing attendants."*

Nursing implications. Analgesic agents, narcotics and nonnarcotics, alcohol, and anesthetics seem to relieve the patient in pain by changing her reaction component to pain. Predominately they do this by alleviating the anxiety or stress present. They do not seem to exert their beneficial influence by altering the transmission of the pain sensation or its original perception.

Nurses similarly seek to help the patient in pain by alleviating the concomitant anxiety and stress and by eliminating minor contributing discomforts. This may be attained through many means.

The *physical environment* of the patient in pain can be modified to reduce and prevent anxiety, fatigue, and stress by elimination of noxious noises, sudden movements and jarring, and strong lights and by maintenance of optimum room temperature, air ventilation, and freedom from strong odors.

A greater degree of personal *physical comfort* can be attained for the patient in pain by early reduction or elimination of new sites of discomfort such as a distending bladder, provoking constipation, or skeletal muscle spasms. A skillfully given partial or complete bath, a skillfully made functional bed, body repositioning, improved skeletal muscle support, and a back rub adapted to the ill individual can relax a patient who is rigid and taut with pain. It is wise to tell the patient what is going to be done, its sequence, and its intended effect. Economy of movements and time is essential for all physical movements and manipulations on the patient in pain. In no other instance does the nurse "talk" more effectively through her hands. This nonverbal communication by the nurse best answers the nonverbal language of pain in its most stress-laden period. (The unsure, unpracticed, or apprehensive nurse is poor medicine. Her activity is *not nursing* for the patient in pain.)

Through these and other physical ministrations, the patient in pain receives *emotional comfort.* Through hands, concern for another is expressed, and care, assurance, and safety are extended. The nonverbal language of the nurse is often the dominant influence for the patient. (The nurse who verbally reassures but who cannot or does not provide physical comfort creates a burden of inconsistent actions. By word and inference she extends help to the patient that often never materializes or is inadequate to the patient's expectation.)

Intellectual comfort is extended to the patient in pain when a nurse tries to answer her questions or refers them personally to the doctor, explains unknown words, rephrases misunderstood conversation fragments, and seeks to explain "reasons" for the many unknowns in the life of a patient. For instance, a nurse

---

*Lemon, Henry M.: Control of pain in metastatic cancer, Journal of Chronic Diseases **4**:84, 1956.

recognizes that some patients are more fearful of accepting medications that mask or eliminate the "danger signal" of pain than of bearing the pain itself. Such patients require more "information" in order to achieve reduction of anxiety and to derive benefit from a medication than those patients who expect pain relief quickly and leave its underlying problem to the doctor.

To successfully achieve any measure of nursing a vital *nurse-patient relationship* must exist. The nurse extends goodwill toward the patient and seeks to understand her, even as she seeks to know her own feelings of pain in the presence of this patient. The latter is essential since the nurse's own values may honor or deny the verbal expression of pain, and she may feel unconcern, anger, or disgust with those who are different. With identification and understanding of the patient's differentness, uncensored communication becomes easier, and both patient and nurse are encouraged to more adequate and accurate expression and interpretation. Tension and anxiety are reduced in such an atmosphere. To the patient the hospital becomes a safer and more therapeutic place.

The administration of an *analgesic* for the alleviation of pain is indicated last, not because it is always the last given, but rather because it is believed that its *full* effectiveness is dependent on the manner in which it is given in conjunction with the other nursing ministrations and relationships mentioned. Nursing measures can directly minimize pain. When nursing accompanies the administration of an analgesic, it augments the effectiveness of the medication. Just as every medication holds an unknown therapeutic benefit beyond its pharmaceutic properties, so a sensitive quality of nursing can influence the patient's pain experience beyond the *seemingly* simple procedures themselves.

RECOMMENDED READINGS FOR STUDENTS

Crowley, Dorothy M.: Pain and its alleviation, Berkeley, 1962, University of California Press.

MacBryde, Mitchell Cyril, editor: Signs and symptoms: Applied pathologic physiology and clinical interpretation, Philadelphia, 1964, J. B. Lippincott & Co.

Melzack, Roland: The perception of pain, Scientific American **204**:41-49, 1961.

Petrovich, Donald V.: A survey of painfulness concepts, Journal of Clinical Psychology **14:** 288-291, 1958.

Ruesch, Jurgen, and Kees, Weldon: Non-verbal communication: Notes on the visual perception of human relations, Berkeley, 1964, University of California Press.

Zborowski, Mark: Cultural components in responses to pain. In Jaco, E. Gartly, editor: Patients, physicians and illness, New York, 1958, Free Press of Glencoe, Inc., pp. 256-268.

RECOMMENDED READINGS FOR INSTRUCTORS AND THE
EXCEPTIONAL STUDENT

Beecher, Henry K.: Measurement of subjective responses, New York, 1959, Oxford University Press.

Buytendijk, F. J. J.: Pain, its modes and functions, Chicago, 1962, University of Chicago Press. (Translated by Eda O'Shiel.)

Gerard, Ralph W.: The physiology of pain, Annals of the New York Academy of Sciences **86:**6-12, 1960.

Chapter 3

The preoperative patient

The periods of time for the surgical patient (preoperative, operative, post-operative, and convalescent) are as changeable for the patient, and therefore for those trying to understand her, as the constant shifting of desert sands. She has direction and then is directionless; she is fearful and then hopeful; she is dependent and yet independent in the course of her illness. If optimum healing is to occur, the patient and those in contact with her are interdependent. Within these periods of time, the patient needs to receive that which makes it possible for her to help herself. If the helping professions are to be able to give to her, she must be able to give to them her trust and her willingness to receive from others. In order to help they must rely on her ability to be both dependent and independent.

Recent studies have substantiated the patient-known truism that the hospital is neither a neutral environment nor a passive one and that the helping-healing professional workers are neither neutral nor passive entities in the healing process. Schottstaedt has clinically measured the amount and duration of metabolic and electrolyte imbalance incurred in patients within a "therapeutic setting" when nurses ignored patients or reprimanded them. The greatest fluctuation in sodium and potassium balances involving all patients in the unit was generated by staff nurses who had been provoked by a nursing administrative edict. Patients felt the tension of the nurses; some felt they were personally hostile to them during this time and reacted not only by individual overt behaviors but also by rather similar internal responses to an unfriendly and stressful environment.*

No one cares to think of herself as one who harms another or who is a deterrent to another's progress or inherent potential. The act of nursing cannot contain this element, for its very function is nurture. However, as the instruments

---

*Schottstaedt, William W., Pinsky, Ruth H., Mackler, David, and Wolf, Stewart: Sociologic, psychologic and metabolic observations on patients in the community of a metabolic ward, American Journal of Medicine 25:248-257, 1958.

through which the act of nursing is given, nurses can give good or ill, can enhance or inhibit, and can help to create or can help to destroy. When the negative aspect is given by a nurse, *nursing* is not given. Yet the patient receives, and she responds, interacts, and reacts within the therapeutically positive and negative atmosphere in a manner that is unique to her.

Within the surgical periods are many possibilities for a negative environment from the patient's standpoint. Such an environment will not help her and may actually hinder her in achieving those tasks that are necessary for her safety and recovery. Since an environment that is nonbeneficial to the family will hold harmful elements for the patient by direct spread, any consideration of the patient must also include the family. It is toward increased recognition and sensitivity of the patient's environment and the role of the nurse within it that these chapters on preoperative and postoperative patients are devoted.

The surgical patient has four major tasks to perform. One of these is a preoperative task. *The patient and her family must prepare themselves emotionally to cope with the stresses of hospitalization and surgery and the illness itself. How well they handle this and how they are helped to cope with the presurgery period in their lives will influence the physical course of the immediate and later surgical periods.*

PREDIAGNOSIS PERIOD

Velpeau, professor of surgery at the University of Paris, in 1839 spoke of "surgery and pain, the inseparables." A few years later the first successful abdominal surgery was performed in Kentucky, with the removal of a large ovarian tumor. Its success was attributed to the anesthetic used. Within the same period of time, Sims, relying upon anesthetic agents to adequately relax patients, performed the first successful vaginal plastic procedure. The advent of anesthesia and analgesics made surgery and surgical pain separable.

Yet when the patient today faces the prospects of her own operation, the *fears* of pain, death, and the surgical procedure still are inseparable. The patient who has noted frightening physical symptoms must now weigh the threatening consequences of a disease entity against uncertain life-threatening or life-restoring surgery. The surgery itself holds peculiar consequences for the woman contemplating a gynecologic operation. As restorative surgery it may ensure a "cure" of a particular disease. However, as a result, she may face the possible loss of certain parts of the body that mean to her or to her husband incompleteness or feared loss of femininity. Another threat may be the anesthesia itself, a fear of being put to sleep, which arouses the fear of not awakening. She may fear surgical pain, but she may fear unconsciousness more, for that means the inability to know and to be in control.

These fears may arise and coexist as the patient increasingly or suddenly becomes aware of symptoms or signs that indicate that perhaps she is not well. Abnormal bleeding, abdominal pain, vaginal discharge, abdominal enlargement, or protrusion of pelvic organs through the introitus will prompt the patient to eventually seek a doctor. But what doctor? Sometimes she initially seeks the confidence and counsel of a friend or neighbor who is a nurse. If the nurse is accessible to her friends and neighbors in this role, accentuating fears and needless delays often can be averted in early stages of gynecologic symptoms.

Since nurses often are asked to recommend doctors, the responsibility inherent in the recommendation should be recognized and not dodged. What are the criteria that guide her decision? How knowledgeable is she of medical-surgical specialists? Should she refer the patient with "seeming" gynecologic problems to the generalist, the internist, or directly to a gynecologist? Does she have sufficient knowledge of the symptoms and their possible implications so that she will neither unduly frighten nor unsafely reassure the patient? What are the criteria guiding her decision of *which doctor* for *this patient?* Does she recognize the personal factors that may influence her decisions? If nursing is really a profession, then she will be asked to be a nurse and to nurture at times other than the eight hours when she wears her uniform and even years after "retirement" from her profession. Despite her own changed self-image, to a neighbor or friend contemplating the presence of illness, she is a nurse. Whether she extends help at this time, how, and in what way or whether she refuses help directly by noninvolvement or indirectly by noncommitment, the patient's response to her illness will be influenced in some way. *When* the patient seeks a doctor, *whom* she seeks, and *how* she is prepared for the visit is often directly related to the advice and concern of others or the lack of it; often these others are nurses, or could be.

PHYSICAL EXAMINATION PERIOD

Every individual becomes self-concerned at the time of a physical examination, even a routine one. Thus the gynecologic patient relies heavily on feelings of goodwill and evidences of regard for her by the nurse and the personnel in the doctor's office, even before the examination. Because of her anxiety and overconcern with self, she is easily hurt or angered by any interpretation of unconcern toward her. Indications of impatience or unfriendliness in office personnel or the anxious feelings imparted by a harried office environment may augment a patient's mounting anxiety. She may begin to evaluate the doctor whom she has not seen by the success or failure of her interpersonal contacts with those who represent him in his office. This initial experience therefore may either enhance confidence and trust or may begin to dissipate it in proportion to the patient's interpretation of her physical and interpersonal environment. She may also interpret the interpersonal relationships of other patients with the personnel within the office environment.

Office personnel within this environment therefore are much more than "schedulers" and "expediters" of that schedule. It is important that office personnel maintain sensitivities to the ongoing "temperature" of the waiting room, so that when tensions rise they may be dealt with individually. Since an individual's perception of any situation narrows in the presence of stress and loses many aspects of accuracy, misunderstandings and unpleasant personal encounters require interpretation to those who wait laden with anxieties. Confidence and trust or distrust and mounting dread are also generated in the waiting room between patient and patient.

Alone with her thoughts in a waiting room, the patient may worry about an unknown procedure, feel embarrassment concerning the scheduled examination, or experience mounting anxiety as the time draws closer when she will find out the meaning of her symptoms. She may even feel she "shouldn't have bothered to come" and wish she could retreat. Fear of the outcome of a diagnosis, fear of the consequences of illness, and perhaps fear of the therapy itself abound within any waiting room.

Some doctors and their office personnel have found that FM music, judiciously monitored according to the waiting-room population and set at a low volume, seems to reduce unnecessary waiting-room jitters and tempers.

It is because of these fears and self-preoccupations that some patients are often forgetful in the examining room and seemingly are unable to comprehend simple directions in preparation for the examination. A patient may "forget" which articles of clothing are to be removed; she may "forget" that she was also requested to void, *or* she may not have understood the word "void" and is too embarrassed and/or excited to ask. She may be fearful that the doctor will walk in as she is voiding. She may be too embarrassed to leave a specimen in plain view for the doctor and may try to hide it. She may spill it and thereby suffer further embarrassment and increasing anxiety prior to the examination. These are clues that this patient's anxiety makes it difficult for her to handle or cope with new directions, simple tasks, and usually performed manipulative dressing skills. She needs help when the anxious head cannot remember, the hands cannot coordinate, and the leaden feet stumble getting upon the examining table. But what adult woman or adolescent girl could possibly ask for help in undressing or help for performance of a simply given direction without also being embarrassed and losing self-respect? If the nurse "seems" aloof, impatient, or hurried, the patient is further inhibited in her furtive seeking to do the right thing and in her unspoken desire to ask help and clarification of what is expected of her.

When an interpersonal communication fails, the volume of the message is often increased and each repetition of the request or direction becomes increasingly louder, though the content of the message may remain the same. It remains obscure even though loud and the patient remains confused. Tension can be reduced if one-sided feelings of helplessness and depreciation can be eliminated. The patient can be relieved of the embarrassment and frustration of misunderstanding if the nurse or other individuals with the patient can admit to themselves and verbally to the patient that messages are frequently garbled by *both* sender and receiver. This places both nurse and patient in the equal position of desiring to understand and openly communicate with one another. Under these conditions communication is usually more appropriately geared to the situation of stress; that is, more words or expressions are attempted that can be comprehended by both patient and nurse, and the sentence structure is shortened to meet the changed need of an anxious patient with a reduced attention span. Fragmented sentences and dangling subjects are frequently encountered in attempted verbal communication by an individual experiencing stress. It is as though she must conserve herself and must draw on all reserves to handle the situation. This means economy of action and emotion as well as speech.

During and after the examination, when the findings are explained to this patient, supplemental help by the nurse as the liaison between the doctor and patient is sometimes necessary. It may help the patient to have an "interpreter" who can expand her verbal communication, break down the doctor's language to meet this situation, and to anticipate her unasked questions. Unless the doctor recognizes the fact that all individuals revert to unique forms of nonverbal communication during stressful situations and accepts the fact that some patients can feel stress in his presence, the patient-doctor communication will fail for lack of comprehension. As a member of the same sex and as one whose status is lower than the doctor's in the patient's eyes, the nurse is more accessible and approachable to the patient. Her function as interpreter and mediator is a very important one.

Some patients come to the doctor expecting to hear that an operation is indicated. This may be based upon painful, fearful, or embarrassing symptoms. A patient with endometriosis may have pain so great by the time operation is proposed by the doctor that its relief-giving promises are accepted by the patient as, "It's worth it." The patient with uterine prolapse may have been living with the condition for a long time, embarrassed and fearful of its consequences, and at the same time embarrassed and fearful of its continued presence. Urinary incontinence, dribbling, and soiling associated with the prolapse make the condition disagreeable enough for her to welcome surgical intervention at any age.

The patient with polyps or fibroids may have had abnormal bleeding, weakness, or a fear of carcinoma that brings her to the doctor. She may dread the examination since it might substantiate her own fearful diagnosis.

Some patients may come only for a routine examination. They may be symptom free or have only slight symptoms such as weight gain around the middle which they may have attributed to middle age, backache, one or two unconnected incidents of spotting, or a difference in the menstrual cycle which they could almost ignore. At the time of examination the disease entity will be diagnosed and perhaps operation immediately prescribed. Patients who have had slight symptoms or no symptoms will little comprehend at the time the necessity for and the reality of an impending surgical procedure. This patient has not even thought of herself as ill. Often such a patient will be very anxious and uncertain. To her there is a subtle danger involved. She is asked to rely solely on her doctor's interpretation of personal danger. She is therefore dependent on a strong doctor-patient relationship. This is in no little measure enhanced by a strong nurse-patient relationship, both before the examination and after the examination, and may be further enhanced by nurse-nurse communication from the office to the hospital. Communication between the nurse in the doctor's office and the hospital unit to which the patient will be admitted can serve as a bond of continuity and provide greater understanding for this patient when she is admitted to the hospital unit.

Some patients may delay in coming to the doctor. These patients are of all social classes, all economic groups, and all professions. It is said that some of the worse offenders are nurses and doctors. Studies of patients who delay in seeking medical attention indicate that these patients are fearful of the illness and seem unable to initiate any activity, are fearful that the treatment will cause inordinate pain, are fearful of harsh treatment, are unable to ask for help, or are unwilling to be dependent, since they view sickness as a sign of weakness and inadequacy.*

Whatever the reason, patient delay is little tolerated by the doctor or by the nurse. It is reflected by an attitude of, "I have no sympathy for anyone who won't try to help herself." It is born of the frustration of the healing professions when they consider the expensive waste of time and their inability to provide the patient much help. Frustration begets anger, and anger begets scorn or depreciation—directed usually, if possible, at the one who aroused the initial frustration. Undoubtedly the patient and her family also feel the guilt of delay or the remorse of delay and therefore need the freely extended help of the healing professions, rather than judgment. This patient and family also require special recognition and understanding by the hospital personnel. Unless the nurse in the office relays this to personnel on the admitting hospital unit, hospital nurses are unaware of what guilt and anguish a patient brings with her as she is admitted. All patients are different! Not only is it important for admitting nurses to know the patient who has delayed treatment but it is also important for the nurse to recognize her in the postoperative period. How *will* this patient get along postoperatively? Will she fight or will she give up? Will she be overwhelmed and unable to ask for help? Her preoperative interpersonal relationships will influence her postoperative response.

PREOPERATIVE HOSPITALIZATION PERIOD

The patient's actual hospitalization is only one more experience added to the others she has had because of this illness. When she enters the hospital, she has had at least most of the following experiences: she has become aware of an unusual feeling or sign, sometimes a very fear-arousing one; she has interpreted this with a gradual or a sudden realization that she is not physically well, that she indeed could be very ill; she has had to decide when and how to ask for help, perhaps to choose a new doctor, to actually make an appointment and to keep

---

*Cobb, Beatrix, Clark, R. Lee, Jr., McGuire, Carson, and Howe, C. D.: Patient-responsible delay of treatment in cancer: A social psychological study, Cancer 7:920-925, 1954. See also Titchener, James L., and Levine, Maurice: Surgery as a human experience, New York, 1960, Oxford University Press, pp. 154-159.

that appointment; she has had to share her anxieties with some members of her family, even though this may have meant adding fresh worries to another ill or financially stressed individual; she may have carried her illness anxieties alone; she has accepted the diagnosis of illness and the prescribed surgical treatment; she has made arrangements for hospitalization, for financing, for her absence from the family unit, for substitute working arrangements, and for substitute civic responsibilities. She has put her personal house in order and she has said her good-byes. This implies her ability to make decisions, to organize and control her life, and to interact with others. She is therefore not helpless or irresponsible as she enters the hospital. Often, however, she *is* an emotionally and physically fatigued individual who is also physically ill. She is an adult in whom feelings of dependence and subjection to the power of others are disquieting. She is a normal adult in whom a reaction to these feelings normally takes the form of fight and resistance or passive capitulation.

The patient and her family

The patient, family, and nurse relationship is created at such an anxiety-laden time. They may learn about each other faster and easier since they need one another. They may talk through one another. They may interpret what one another has to say. Through a reduction of the family's helplessness and noninvolvement in the hospitalization may be fostered an optimum patient-family, patient-nurse, and family-nurse relationship. The significance of this to the patient and the family is acceptance and goodwill on the part of the hospital staff, which further encourages and improves communication in all directions.

The importance of the family throughout the illness can never be underestimated. The attitudes and actions of one member influence the other. The family evaluates the hospital milieu, the friendliness and safeness of the hospital, and the people who will care for the member of their family. They seek reassurances of the personnel through their responses and actions. However, the family seldom receives concentrated or selective contact with those people who will be most concerned with the patient, and the anxiousness of the family becomes manifest in signs of restlessness, quiet withdrawal, overtalking, or demanding. The nurse can minimize this through a giving relationship not only to the patient but also to the family. She can protect the environment so the family will not be so fearful and anxious. She can enhance the environment by bringing the family closer to the patient. This means inclusion of the family *with* the patient in the hospitalization. A German proverb says, "Geteiler Schmerz ist halber Schmerz," which can be translated as "Half the suffering is removed when it is shared."

Why can the hospital nurse not share some of the unknowns and strangenesses of the hospital with the patient and her family? Can she remember her own feelings of awkwardness and dependence upon others in new situations? Particularly can she remember her own feelings within a new hospital setting? If so, she will find ways to help both the patient and family to know what to expect, what is expected of them, what to expect of others, and who those others are within the setting of the hospital.

Sharing with the family and patient that they in turn may share with one another will include some orientation by the nurse.

Orienting patient and family to plans, schedules, and hospital personnel prior to operation. The nurse can help the patient and family in identification of uniforms worn by aides, orderlies, interns, residents, medical clerks, laboratory technicians, anesthesiologist, student nurse, practical nurse, graduate nurse, social worker, and hospital chaplain. She can supplement the doctor's explanation of the tests and procedures that will be carried out prior to operation. She can reassure them of the periodic rounds of the attending and house staff doctors and the nurses and their accessibility to her. She can dispel possible fears of night noises and night lights such as flashlights.

Orienting patient and family to recovery room. The nurse can orient the patient and the family to the recovery room, its staffing, what kinds of patients are sent there, its availability to the family, its location, how the family will be notified that the patient is there, and approximately how long the patient might be there. The families will be relieved to know when the doctor will see them, *where* he will see them, and how they can find him. Both the patient and family are acutely dependent upon the knowledge and experience of strangers during this period. Anxiousness will be lessened by advance identification of the recovery period and knowing who will be there. Will there be nurses and personnel they already know or new ones? If the nurse knows them, the family and patient can begin to feel they know them through her.

Orienting patient and family to early postoperative period. Other unknowns or the activities expected of the patient postoperatively can also be shared with the patient. These include the frequent turning of the patient with assistance, the relationship of pain with movement, the best ways to move and to roll, the importance of moving the legs freely and frequently, and the purpose and importance of deep breathing and coughing. Most important, she can show the family how the patient will help and *how* the family can help when the nurse thinks such assistance is needed. This immediately helps both the patient and family by soliciting their participation before the operation and includes them in an active participating role during the postoperative period. It also obviates later fears and apprehensions due to unknowns. For example, the patient will be requested to cough frequently. However, to a family, coughing is associated with infection, and therefore, the coughing patient may seem to them to have a complication.

Before the operation is also the time to have the patient experience what abdominal muscles are strained when she coughs and therefore where and how she can splint and guard her abdominal incision postoperatively when she coughs. She then becomes a knowledgeable and more assured patient who works toward her own recovery with the professional assistance of the helping-healing professions.

She becomes interdependent with them in the common goal of recovery. Her family will also exhibit less anxiety because they experience fewer of the unknowns of the situation. They too feel involved and accepted, and feeling this way will benefit the patient.

The patient in the hospital

The newly admitted surgical patient is considered the "most well" of all patients on the unit, at least the most able to take care of herself. Usually she is expected to conform to the hospital customs without really knowing what they are. She has feelings of awkwardness and helplessness in the new situation. She has varying amounts of free time and often becomes the floor pacer within her own room or the hallway. This is the period when she becomes acquainted with her new environment through her own eyes and through other patient contacts, her room-mate, or other pacers. By these means, she gains a positive or negative orientation to the hospital. She sees previews of future days as a surgical patient. She has informal contacts with personnel, seeing and hearing them in relation to herself and others, and she projects herself as a helpless patient with this personnel.

During this waiting period the patient may be very receptive for new learning and these may become important teaching moments. Through a foreknowledge of the patient from the office nurse and through her own observations and knowledge of this patient, the nurse may preplan periods of time when teaching would be most receptively received, or it may arise spontaneously at an opportune time. Her teaching could include at least these three areas: (1) an introduction to the hospital vocabulary—the medical terminology that is used by hospital personnel with the assumption that it is understood, (2) a foreknowledge of the information required by the gynecologist and/or the anesthesiologist to expand their knowledge of the patient's preoperative condition and (3) a foreknowledge of that preparation that has as its aim protection of the patient for the eventual operative procedure.

Giving patient an introduction to hospital vocabulary. Every nurse secretly recalls that time when the terminology heard and used in the hospital setting was strange and new and completely unintelligible to her: the time when hospital conversation flowed about her ears like a foreign language and she wondered, "What was that all about?" Medical terminology is confusing, unintelligible, and often ambiguous to almost all hospitalized patients. It provides another stressor to an already anxious patient who must now try to interpret its meaning. It is compounded stress for the hospitalized patient who has a hearing impairment, to one who is young, or to one who is very old.

A recent study* has validated the communications plight of the patient and shows that most patients lack the knowledge and understanding of words commonly used in their presence which medical personnel "assume" they comprehend. Some

---

*Samora, Julian, Saunders, Lyle, and Larson, Richard F.: Medical vocabulary knowledge among hospital patients, Journal of Health and Human Behavior **2:**83-92, 1961.

of these words are void, stool, I.V., suction, catheter, dressing, and suture. Probably few nurses, doctors, or medical personnel knew these words before beginning their education. Yet we all expect patients to know them. This study emphasizes the anxieties associated with misunderstanding or lack of understanding on the part of the patient, especially when everyone acts as though she should know what is being said. Because a patient has been hospitalized before or because a patient is well educated is no valid reason to assume that she has superior comprehension of hospital and medical terminology. To the preceding terms could also be added the directives that are given to but seldom defined for patients. These would include "bed rest," "bathroom privileges" (which seems to vary from hospital to hospital and from doctor to doctor), and "N.P.O." or "hold." Seldom are patients told exactly what these words or abbreviations mean. Patients rarely know how much activity is permitted or denied them with bed rest, bathroom privileges, or ward privileges. What *is* the difference between all three? When a patient is on a "hold breakfast," does she understand she cannot eat, so that she will not feel neglected and forgotten when her meal does not arrive? "Oversights" are often responsible for needless fear, lack of understanding, and lack of confidence in the treatment or care that the patient thinks she should be receiving. It may mean to her that she is committed to an "unsafe" environment. If so, it is detrimental to her.

> A patient was told, "We're going to get some electrolytes on you." The patient accepted the statement with silent wonder and waited from 8 A.M. rounds until evening for a heat cradle such as her roommate had once had. She felt vulnerable throughout the day because *someone* was not carrying out the doctor's orders. She equated it with lack of safe care and she felt forgotten and denied. After the word "electrolyte" was finally explained to her, she had an immediate reaction of facial flushing, she felt "stupid" and later felt resentment that she had been made to worry for nothing and that her "ignorance" was exposed. The patient could have been spared this entire day of destructive processes.

An even more serious misunderstanding was the following:

> The patient had had an abdominal hysterectomy. Almost two weeks later she was startled as she conversed with her doctors, "I thought you were just taking out my uterus. I didn't know you were taking out my womb." She cried because she had not realized what they were going to do.

This patient had not fully realized what was going to happen to her because she did not comprehend the language. Sensitivity and awareness of this problem by the hospital personnel is the first step. The second, of necessity, is being able to know the subject so well that they can break down large words into small ones and use accurate examples. During the course of personal interactions with the patient in the preoperative period, many opportunities are afforded to help the patient know some of these words of hospital expression and to evaluate the patient's comprehension of what has been told her by others.

Giving patient foreknowledge of preparations for operation. The preparations required by the gynecologist or anesthesiologist to expand their knowledge of the patient's preoperative condition usually includes history taking and laboratory work such as urinalysis, blood tests, and chest x-ray examinations. While patients usually are assured that this work has been ordered for them, they often have no idea why. A chest x-ray study prior to gynecologic procedures may seem highly unrelated. Questions may not be asked and patients wonder and fear that many things are being kept from them. Since adequate renal function and adequate oxygenation of blood are essentials for maximum postoperative recovery after the trauma of surgery, the patient should feel reassurances that such examinations are performed preoperatively for her safety.

Possible additions to the routine laboratory work may involve a barium enema or an intravenous pyelogram. The patient usually enters the hospital knowing that she will have these, but since the time this was explained to her in the doctor's office, she may now have questions about them. Some patients are hesitant to question the doctor, particularly when he has explained things to them at a previous time. They feel they are taking up his time, they may be ashamed to admit their lack of knowledge after his explanation, or they may be ashamed to admit their apprehension.

X-ray procedures are seldom discussed with the patient in the hospital. The patient is taken to just one more strange area in the hospital and undergoes one more strange procedure. Sometimes a patient has received information about x-ray procedures from friends, family, or roommates having had similar experiences, and unfortunately, unless the nurse is very familiar with x-ray techniques, these informants usually can tell the patient more than she can. For this reason alone, it should be urged that all nurses become acquainted with all other departments where their patients are taken for tests so they may know and understand what the patients experience when the nurse is no longer with them. Then nurses will better understand the responses of a patient when she returns to the unit.

For the x-ray department, this means that the nurse, as a visitor, will be aware of how that department looks and thereby be sensitive to how it would appear to the elderly patient, the very young patient, or the very anxious patient. She will be aware of the discomforts experienced, the long waiting between films, where they wait, and what they see as they wait. She will know of the hard unyielding table and its effect on the arthritic patient, the elderly patient, or the cachectic patient. She will be aware of the embarrassments of the patient who is not able to retain the barium given as an enema and of the perhaps inadequate draping in a rather public department. She will have an understanding of the possible scary aspects of x-ray examinations, a sometimes totally black room, a moving and tilting x-ray table, a large, formidable machine, the clicking of the machine, the lights that flash, and the bells. She will therefore be more sensitive to the old and young patients who go to the x-ray department. She will realize the isolation of the patient while the examination is performed and the invisible, intangible quality of roentgen rays, combined with the stories of radiation dangers that lay people now read.

In addition to being acquainted with the x-ray department, it would be desirable for nurses to be acquainted with the personnel and what they are like as people. A nurse so oriented can anticipate and help her patient with answers and with information that the patient would not think of asking. She can make the situation of x-ray examination or any diagnostic test less stressful and avoid surprise by preparing the patient for the events to occur. She can prepare the patient to meet the new personnel, perhaps calling some of them by name. She can give simple explanations about the technique that may clarify doubts in the mind of the patient.

A simple explanation means reducing the subject to basics, not a minimum of words. For example, to tell a patient who is going to have an intravenous pyelogram (I.V.P.), "They'll put a dye in your arm, and then they'll take an x-ray," arouses many more fears than the patient ever could have thought of herself. Rather, it means that the nurse must be sure of her vocabulary and the patient's level of comprehension. Does the patient know the relationship of the kidney, ureter, and bladder and the relationship of the kidney and bladder to the uterus and ovaries? Does she know all of these words? And the word "x-ray": really, what is it? The following account is a good example of an explanation to the patient.*

> It is an invisible ray capable of going through paper, wood, soft skin or tissue, or organs such as the stomach or kidney, but it is not able to go through heavy or dense substances such as bone or some metals, for example, lead. If the rays are directed through the body onto a film, the latter may be developed similarly to photographic film and viewed as a picture, showing the dense substances such as bone or metal. Soft organs such as kidneys will therefore not show on an x-ray film without special techniques. There are dyes that are opaque to roentgen rays which can be used to visualize organs such as the kidneys. Such dyes are called radiopaque.

For the next step, the patient will need additional information.

> All blood in the body goes through little tufts of blood vessels in the kidney, where all the wastes are taken out of the blood and also some water if your body doesn't need it. This forms urine. If a special radiopaque dye is put into a blood vessel, it travels along with the blood until it comes to the kidney, where it is considered a waste product and is removed. Within the urine, it then goes into the ureters or connecting tubes and thence to the urinary bladder. If an x-ray beam is directed at the kidney while the dye is being removed, the opaqueness of the dye creates an image on the film, and the functional position of the kidney (that part of the kidney that the doctor wants to see) can be clearly seen. This is called an intravenous pyelogram or I.V.P. To prepare for this test you will be asked to drink two glasses of water, and some dye will be injected into one of the veins of your arm with a syringe and needle. The dye will not color your skin and will not stay in your body any longer than the time it takes to have the x-ray film taken.

Similar details are necessary in explaining the barium enema examination and preparations for that test.

The example given may be reduced or expanded according to the manner in

---

*See also X-ray . . . and you, New York, no date, Eastman Kodak Co., Medical Division.

which the communication is received by the patient. It would also be altered according to the recent experiences of the patient with x-ray tests or perhaps a recent experience within the clinical unit that makes this information more or less acceptable.

Giving patient information concerning preparations necessary for patient protection. The patient may be told about the residue-free meal and the restrictions on food and fluid prior to operation. This forestalls emesis during operation and minimizes it afterward. The patient or family who understands why the light supper is given will be less fearful of the patient being weak the next day because of an insufficient supper. They will also be less inclined to sneak in a ham sandwich to the patient that night or the next morning to supplement the restricted hospital fare. The nurse can explain that preoperative enemas lessen intestinal loading and therefore ensure greater surgical safety.

The lay public is well aware of infection. Through friends, relatives, neighbors, and articles in national magazines, staphylococcus infections and hospitals are closely associated. Most often it is hospital personnel who have their heads in the sand and say it is not so. Therefore, any patient will be most assured to recognize the precautions that minimize the quantity of skin bacteria prior to operation. These include shaving body and pubic hair, a bath with special soaps, and perhaps a preoperative vaginal suppository or douche.

Although the patient may accept the necessity of all of these preparations, they are not without embarrassment to her. Whether she is receiving them for the first time or the hundredth time, she may fear the danger of soiling the bed when she is given her enema or douche, and she feels embarrassment. She may feel unnatural, naked, and ashamed during the skin preparation. All of these procedures, routine as they are to the nurse and hurried as she may be as she does them, exist to the patient as one more anxiety. The patient may react by being more withdrawn, by chattering, or by becoming more confused by simple directions.

Peplau has said, "Even though the patient has discussed it with [her] surgeon, when [she] comes face to face with the operations preparatory to surgical intervention new feelings may arise and need to be worked through as . . . [she is] prepared for the operation."* This often is the time the patient really begins to express her feelings. She may do so by beginning as one patient did: "When will they take my teeth out? Will anyone see me?" When she sensed adequate concern and understanding by the nurse to these lead questions, she was able to continue and express the deeper and more difficult issues that troubled her.

The married woman patient is often worried by the degree of her self-concern and her introspection at this time. She is concerned for her family and their welfare, but she is more and more anxious about herself, and she feels guilt. Anne Morrow Lindbergh has described a woman thusly, "All her instinct as a woman—

---

*Peplau, Hildegard E.: Interpersonal relations in nursing, New York, 1952, G. P. Putnam's Sons, p. 67.

the eternal nourisher of children, of men, of society—demands that she give. . . . She wants perpetually to spill herself away."*

When the patient is concerned about her own welfare, she cannot give freely. When she cannot give to her family, she feels anxious. During the preoperative period she has a greatly increased need for the love and concern of others. When a person is more concerned with herself, she needs most the evidences of others' love. The amount required and demanded depends upon the previous relationships. Therefore, that patient who has had close relationships and warm affections will continue to feel assured that she will receive it even though ill and will, to a lesser degree, withdraw into herself to maintain herself.

Anesthesia remains a big fear. Usually on the eve of operation the patient has received a visit from the anesthesiologist. Afterward the patient may ask the nurse questions. She may ask questions about books or articles she has read on anesthesia or stories she has heard from friends or relatives. It is therefore urged that a nurse have more information about anesthesia at her fingertips than any lay person. One book on anesthesia is suggested as reference reading in the chapter bibliography. This book was expressly written to dispel the fears usually associated with anesthesia by explaining the subject in simple, nontechnical but informative language. Books available to the lay public as well as articles currently appearing in most national magazines warrant constant review and evaluation, so that nurses may intelligently supplement, interpret, and understand some of the information and ideas acquired by patients.

OPERATING ROOM PERIOD OF THE CONSCIOUS PATIENT

Preparation of the patient may have been excellent in the clinical area. It all may be undone by the environment immediately prior to the operation if patients hear themselves referred to as "the gynecology case for 10 o'clock" or as "Dr. Jones' patient for 10 o'clock." For the first time since her admission to the hospital, this patient may fear a lack of identity. "Do they really know who I am, and who my doctor is?" She is more helpless now than she has ever been since she stepped into the hospital. She is flat on her back on a stretcher, perhaps feeling a little woozy because of the medication given her a short while before, and looking *up* at whoever hesitates long enough to peer down at her. She is completely dependent and very passive.

An eighteenth century court physician once gave the following advice:

'Tis customary to send to the Patient's Chamber (some time before the Chirurgeon comes) a Servant to dispose all things in order; but frequently, by the quantity of bits of Linnen which they cut, the heaps of Lint which they make, and the spreading shew of numerous Instruments, they strike Fear and Terror into the Mind of the Patient, by giving him a cruel Idea of the Operation which they are going about. I would that the Chirurgeons would not shew themselves to their Patients, 'til the Moment appointed

---

*Lindbergh, Anne Morrow: Gift from the sea, New York, 1955, Pantheon Books, Inc., Chapter 3.

for the Operation. . . . I would then have him affable to his Patient, that he encourage and hearten him, that he participate of his Affliction, and promise him to the least Pain possible.*

The patient today appreciates seeing her doctor before operation and also appreciates the closeness of the nurse or the attendant who brings her to the operating room. Yet too often the person who transports the patient may be considered merely a chauffeur who impersonally carries out his function of pushing the stretcher. The patient may be left in a strange area, knowing no one and, as in the eighteenth century, is left to observe preparations or activity prior to someone's operation, perhaps even her own. The clink of instruments as they are arranged on tables, the scrubbing of nurses and doctors, and the wheeling of gas machines are common sights and sounds for the surgical patient in the twentieth century. The positive and negative experiences occurring within this period to the patient in no small degree determine her postoperative course. If any part of the preoperative period has contained situations that the patient has perceived as threatening, depressing, or hopeless, she may draw on precious physiologic and psychologic reserves, which should be conserved for the stresses of the operation itself. It is possible that because of these situations the patient may enter the operating room unprepared, defeated, frightened, or exhausted.

The success of the preoperative period as a preparatory period to the stresses of surgery can be measured by the postoperative course. In particular, the manner of arousal from anesthesia, the amount of nausea and pain, and the quality of wound healing can be *directly* influenced by the success or failure of the presurgical preparation. The nurse's role is a very influential one in this period.

---

*Cited in Ricci, James V.: Development of gynaecological surgery and instruments, Philadelphia, 1949, Blakiston Division, McGraw-Hill Book Co., Inc., p. 191.

RECOMMENDED READINGS FOR STUDENTS

Gregg, Dorothy E.: Anxiety—a factor in nursing care, American Journal of Nursing **52:**1363-1365, 1952.

Kaplan, Stanley: Laboratory procedures as emotional stress, Journal of the American Medical Association **161:**677-681, 1956.

Schottstaedt, William W., Pinsky, Ruth H., Mackler, David, and Wolf, Stewart: Sociologic, psychologic and metabolic observations on patients in the community of a metabolic ward, American Journal of Medicine **25:**248-257, 1958.

Shane, Sylvan M.: Anaesthesia, thief of pain, New York, 1956, Vantage Press.

RECOMMENDED READINGS FOR INSTRUCTORS

Fischer, H. Keith: Emotional problems associated with gynecologic surgery, Clinical Obstetrics and Gynecology **5:**597-614, 1962.

Hayakawa, S. I.: Conditions of success in communication, Bulletin of the Menninger Clinic **26:**225-236, 1962.

Skipper, James K., Tagliacozzo, Daisy L., and Mauksch, Hans O.: Some possible consequences of limited communication between patients and hospital functionaries, Journal of Health and Human Behavior **5:**34-39, 1964.

Titchener, James L., and Levine, Maurice: Surgery as a human experience, New York, 1960, Oxford University Press.

READINGS ACCESSIBLE TO PATIENTS

Davis, Edwina: Medical language made easy, Today's Health **43**(1):34-37, 1965.

Grafton, Samuel: The hidden epidemic, McCall's Magazine, July, 52-53, 125-128, 130, 1961.

Hysterectomy: When it's needed, what it does, Good Housekeeping **160**(1):139, 1965.

Irwin, Theodore: Your life is in their hands, Today's Health **42**(8):30-33, 52-53, 1964.

Naismith, Grace: D and C: Most common operation on women, Today's Health **42**(7):18, 48-50, 1964.

Shane, Sylvan M.: Anaesthesia, thief of pain, New York, 1956, Vantage Press.

Pamphlets

X-ray, the inside story (Robert S. Sherman and John S. Laughlin, consultants), Binghamton, N. Y., no date, American College of Radiology.

X-rays . . . and you, New York, no date, Eastman Kodak Co., Medical Division.

Chapter 4

The postoperative patient

PATTERNS OF RESPONSE TO GYNECOLOGIC PROCEDURES

Following most *minor* gynecologic procedures, patients are ambulated within a few hours. There is little if any pain. Moderate vaginal bleeding is usual for the first few hours and often for a few days after a curettage. Spontaneous voiding is expected. The patient tolerates and enjoys light food a few hours after the procedure. It may be assumed that the period of survival mechanisms after these procedures is short and that the sympathetic nervous system influences soon wane. The convalescent phase of tissue restoration begins. The patient is usually able to go home either on the first or second postoperative day.

Elevation of temperature, pain, or excessive and continued bleeding indicate possible postoperative complications. The presence of such symptoms and the complications that they connote renew the sympathetic nervous system influences. The convalescent course is delayed until the new stressors are reduced and the complication is alleviated.

Major gynecologic procedures entail partial or complete excision of reproductive organs or plastic repair of defects. The removal of an ovary (oophorectomy), a myoma (myomectomy), a uterine tube (salpingectomy), the entire uterus (total or complete hysterectomy), the uterus with tubes and ovaries (hysterectomy with bilateral salpingo-oophorectomy), or the vulva (vulvectomy) are major gynecologic procedures. Repairs of fistulas from the vagina into the bladder (vesicovaginal) or from the vagina into the rectum (rectovaginal), repairs of the anterior or posterior vaginal wall because of a protrusion of the urethra (urethrocele), the bladder (cystocele), or the rectum (rectocele), and the repair of the cul-de-sac because of a protrusion of the intestine (enterocele) are also major gynecologic procedures. In the absence of septic conditions, invasive malignancy, or coexistent chronic diseases such as diabetes or cardiac dysfunctions, the gynecologic patient usually has a rapid and complication-free postoperative course and is discharged from the hospital by the tenth to the twelfth day.

After major gynecologic procedures, vaginal or abdominal, overdistention of the urinary bladder must be avoided. The postoperative patient is sedated and usually receiving intravenous fluid. Seldom does she void spontaneously. Catheterization may be necessary both immediately and in the later postoperative period. This disability may last three to eight days or occasionally longer.

Pain is limited to the incision area and pelvic and lower abdominal regions. It may be severe the first two postoperative days. Narcotics are usually required during this time. The patient's recovery and comfort depend to some extent upon the careful administration of medications. If there is doubt regarding the dose or type of drug, the nurse should obtain immediate medical confirmation consultation. After the third day the pain is much less and simple analgesics usually suffice.

The body temperature may be elevated (up to 102° F.) during the first one or two postoperative days without complications. By the fifth postoperative day the temperature is normal in patients who have had no complications.

Nausea and vomiting are common following anesthesia the first postoperative day, but seldom after that time. The intestinal pattern following pelvic laparotomy is one of protective ileus, with a soft, silent nontender abdomen, and then gradual resumption of intestinal movements, with the urge to defecate occurring about four to five days postoperatively. Enemas or a mild laxative at this time may alleviate the discomfort associated with defecation.

After complete hysterectomy, vaginal bleeding, slight in amount, is frequent during the first few postoperative days.

Vaginal discharge with a foul odor is frequent after complete hysterectomy but should be small in quantity and should clear promptly.

Generally, the patient who has had a vaginal procedure moves in bed with greater ease (the vulvectomy patient excepted) than the patient who has had an abdominal procedure, tolerates fluids and food sooner, and expresses no fear that the wound might lack integrity and might reopen.

The development of postoperative complications is heralded by deviation from the normal pattern. When a patient's temperature rises to a higher level or remains at a high level after the third postoperative day, a complication is indicated. Persistence of a temperature elevation after the fifth day also indicates a complication. Continuous urinary retention, with increase in symptoms and increase in amount of residual urine, is indicative of a urinary tract problem, as is frequency and dysuria. Oliguria suggests renal failure. Anuria may mean renal failure or occluded ureters. Persistent, increasing, or newly developed pain in the pelvis or general abdomen during the postoperative period indicates some complication. The sudden appearance of a cough and chest pain, with or without fever, may be due to respiratory infection or a much more serious complication—pulmonary infarction. Abdominal distention, nausea and vomiting after the first postoperative day, or cramping abdominal pain is indicative of possible gastrointestinal complications.

A thin serous discharge from an abdominal wound and local tenderness suggest wound disruption. Increasing vaginal bleeding or sudden hemorrhage at any stage means a complication. A sudden gush of odoriferous discharge from the vagina usually indicates the existence of an abscess in the vaginal cuff region.

Postoperative infections

The most common postoperative infections are wound infections, urinary tract infections, thrombophlebitis, peritonitis, pelvic cellulitis, vault abscess, and respiratory infections.

Since most postoperative infections can be successfully managed if diagnosed promptly, the importance of alert nursing recognition is emphasized. Early recognition of the problem, followed by prompt diagnosis, culture, and appropriate treatment, which includes antibiotics and surgical drainage when indicated, results in a very high recovery rate.

Wound infections may be anticipated in the markedly obese patient, in the poorly controlled diabetic patient, and in those who have acute or chronic infections either in the genital organs, gastrointestinal or urinary tracts, or lungs. Correction of these problems prior to operation, if possible, is desirable.

Pain or discomfort and a swollen, indurated, tender region in the wound about the fourth or fifth postoperative day usually are the first indications of a wound infection. In a patient with an unexplained fever the wound should always be inspected. If there is drainage, a culture is taken and appropriate antibiotics are employed. *Escherichia coli, Staphylococcus,* and *Streptococcus* are the most common organisms encountered in an infected wound.

Urinary tract infections comprise almost 30% of the postoperative complications. Coliform bacteria are the offending agents in the vast majority, but there is at present a sharp increase in proteus, enterococcus, and staphylococcus infections. Evaluation of the urinary tract prior to gynecologic procedures by urinalysis, urine cultures, cystoscopy, pyelography, and renography may be indicated. Overuse of catheterization as well as delay in catheterization when indicated may lead to these infections. This has been discussed in another section. Symptoms are frequency, urgency, dysuria, and occasionally hematuria. The diagnosis and management of these infections include urine culture, with sensitivity studies, followed by appropriate antibiotic therapy and adequate hydration. Unresponsive infections indicate further investigations such as cystoscopy and pyelography in order to rule out urinary tract injury.

Thrombophlebitis, though an infrequent complication, usually involves only the superficial vessels of the lower extremities, but it may progress to severe thrombosis, multiple emboli, pulmonary infarction, and death. Probably the most effective prophylaxis of thrombophlebitis is early ambulation, which is carried out on the evening of operation or the first postoperative day. During the operative procedure, proper padding of stirrups, utilized in the lithotomy position, and also wrapping of the lower extremities with elastic bandages when varicosities are present are important. Here the operating room personnel can play an important role, since it is they who position the patients for operation. Superficial thrombophlebitis usually responds well to elevation, heat, and antibiotics. Embolic phenomena require more drastic measures such as analgesics (Demerol), oxygen, vagal inhibition (atropine), anticoagulants, and possible surgical procedures such as embolectomy and ligation of the offending vessel or even the inferior vena cava.

Generalized peritonitis or *pelvic cellulitis* may be the result of an obvious infection present at the time of operation, of the development of an infection secondary to the trauma of the surgical procedure, or of damage to the bowel during the operation. It is recognized by increasing pain, high fever, abdominal distention, tenderness, and a "silent" abdomen. Its management involves major problems of fluid and electrolyte balance, paralytic ileus, mechanical bowel obstruction, septicemia, and abscess formation.

Vault abscesses are particularly bothersome problems following total hysterectomy. They form at the vault just above the closed vaginal mucosa. They usually manifest themselves by persistent fever followed by profuse purulent vaginal discharge, usually about a week following operation. If drainage is established, improvement and healing may be anticipated. A pelvic abscess, one that extends beyond the small vault accumulation, requires surgical drainage through the vagina and this usually heals quite readily.

Pneumonitis, bronchopneumonia, and lobar pneumonia are serious postoperative pulmonary infections and are infrequent. Proper aeration of the lungs following operations can be maintained by the nurse with the help of an oxygen therapy unit. Positive pressure breathing may be indicated in those patients in whom respiratory problems are anticipated. For pulmonary infection, antibiotics in addition to the ancillary aeration procedures usually clear up the problem.

Postoperative intestinal problems

Frequent observation during the postoperative period of the lips, tongue, contour of the abdomen, peristaltic sounds, and reports of bowel action are as essential as those of the pulse, blood pressure, and respiration. Probably the most common cause of postoperative nausea or vomiting is the response of the patient to both drugs and anesthesia. The treatment is simple discontinuation of the medication as well as administration of motion sickness drugs. The nurse should note any deviation, since a major problem may occur with great speed. Pain and distention due to small bowel dysfunction usually are of short duration and subside as the large bowel recovers. The use of a rectal tube, abdominal hot packs, or small enemas will frequently bring relief. However, if pain, distention, and vomiting exceed that which is normally expected or are prolonged, true paralytic ileus or mechanical intestinal obstruction must be considered. Peristaltic sounds that are easily heard through a stethoscope are excellent indicators of bowel function. Almost constant peristalsis, particularly in rushes, implies hyperactivity, while silence signifies ileus. Vaginal and rectal examinations may reveal fecal impaction, fissures, thrombosed hemorrhoids, or the characteristic sign of mechanical small bowel obstruction—a dilated empty rectosigmoid.

Small bowel obstruction is usually due to adhesions either to the abdominal incision or to the tissues at the site of the surgical procedure in the pelvis. It may not be possible to distinguish readily between mechanical obstruction and ileus, particularly if obstruction is low and x-ray findings are equivocal. Gastrointestinal suction, restriction of oral intake, plus intravenous fluids are indicated until the diagnosis is more obvious and either operative or nonoperative treatment is instituted.

Postoperative wound dehiscence

Disruption of an abdominal wound or dehiscence, with or without exposure and protrusion of the abdominal contents (evisceration), is rare. Patients who have a smooth convalescence seldom experience dehiscence. This develops more often in those patients in whom there is an increase in intra-abdominal pressure due to coughing, distention, and vomiting; in those in whom there is weakness of tissue, with delayed wound healing; or in those in whom there is a faulty wound closure. The superficial layers give way in turn and ultimately the wound breaks open. If some of the layers hold, actual evisceration does not occur, but a postoperative incisional hernia may result.

The nurse should be alert to the development of a sudden serous or serosanguinous discharge from the incision, for this is an indication that there is disruption of the wound. The patient may also complain of a sudden tearing pain. Bleeding or the drainage of old dark blood may indicate a subcutaneous hematoma rather than complete wound disruption. If any of these signs or symptoms are present, an attempt should be made to prevent further disruption by using large butterfly tapes or abdominal supports such as binders, and any underlying cause of increased intra-abdominal pressure should be alleviated.

If there is vomiting, distention, or paralytic ileus, a gastrointestinal tube should be passed. The use of antibiotics as well as pertussants should be administered for a cough or upper respiratory infection. Treatment is suture of the wound with through and through sutures that are closely spaced and set back 3 to 4 cm. from the edges of the skin and tied over rubber or plastic tubing in order that they will not cut through the wound. The chance of recurrent dehiscence following such treatment is relatively slight, although a postoperative hernia may develop.

Urinary tract injuries

Injury to the ureter is probably the most serious nonlethal risk of pelvic operations. Although all efforts to prevent ureteral injury may be taken, such injuries continue to occur. The occurrence and its serious consequences can be reduced to a minimum by the doctor's careful preoperative appraisal, by adjustment of the operative procedure to the individual patient, and by early recognition and effective therapy when such an injury does occur. Whereas overt ureteral injury usually is recognized and repaired immediately at the time of the operation, it may go unrecognized until leakage of urine occurs during the convalescence. Unilateral injury without development of a fistula may occasionally culminate in a silent autonephrectomy.

Early postoperative anuria following a pelvic operation may be due to either bilateral ureteral ligation or acute renal shutdown. Radioisotope renograms present characteristic tracings that distinguish between the two entities. Full use of the urologic (cystoscopy and retrograde ureteral catheterization) and radiologic (intravenous and retrograde pyelography) procedures is required to make an exact diagnosis.

Unilateral ureteral injury may be manifested in the early postoperative period by severe flank pain and an abdominal mass or an increase in fever with pyelonephritis. Radioisotope renograms will demonstrate varying degrees of ureteral obstruction, and excretory urography and ureteral catheterization will indicate where the injury has occurred. If transection has occurred, urinary extravasation may be seen and the ureter may then be repaired surgically. Development of a ureterovaginal fistula during the convalescence indicates cystoscopic examination and ureteral catheterization and ultimate surgical treatment.

Vesicovaginal fistula, though at one time the most common urinary tract injury, is becoming quite rare. It is usually due to necrosis of the bladder following ligation for control of hemorrhage or may be due to actual injury during the surgical procedure. The patient complains of constant vaginal drainage which has the odor of urine. This type of fistula can be differentiated from a ureteral-vaginal fistula by the insertion of a dye such as methylene blue into the bladder. Its appearance on a clean sponge placed in the vagina indicates a vesicovaginal fistula. Following the diagnosis the patient must be studied by cystoscopy, so that the relationship of the fistula and the ureters may be ascertained. Repair of these fistulas is usually delayed until all signs of inflammation around the fistula have subsided. The fistula may then be closed, usually vaginally or occasionally by an abdominal procedure. After the operation, constant drainage is essential.

CONVALESCENCE

Throughout the period of convalescence the patient has strong inner forces working toward an equilibrium of health. It is useful to consider convalescence in this way, since it emphasizes the magnitude and multitude of dovetailing processes involved in the patient's recovery. It emphasizes the complexities and changes in the patient's internal environment that are continually influenced by the changing forces of her external environment, that is, the physical environment of the hospital and her interpersonal contacts. It emphasizes the interrelationships of the adaptive forces, the reactions of the patient, and others' reactions to her.

Convalescence may be viewed as an integrated sequence of adaptive processes in response to the trauma of operation. These adaptions are biologic, psychologic, and social. The sequences are visibly noted as clinical signs and, according to

Moore,* may be arbitrarily divided into four phases. These phases are called the "phase of injury," "the turning point," "muscular strength," and "fat gain." Expressed through the experience of the patient, these phases might be termed "the lost days," "turning the corner," "stronger every day and back to work," and "I feel my old self again." During the "phase of injury" the task of the patient is *to utilize optimum protective and adaptive mechanisms for survival*. During the later three phases of convalescence the tasks of the patient are *to utilize optimum adaptive and restorative mechanisms for wound healing* and *to prepare for the resumption of her role within the home*. These phases therefore may be reduced to two functional periods: the period of survival mechanisms after the trauma of the operation and the later period of restorative mechanisms. During these phases or periods the function of the helping-healing professions is to help the patient achieve the goals of survival and restoration.

Clinically, the phases of convalescence are seen in some patients as distinct patterns, while in other patients one phase may merge into another with little differentiation. Their duration as well as their distinct characteristics are influenced by many factors. Some of these are the extent of the operative trauma, the physical and psychologic stamina of the patient, the amount of blood loss, the fluid balance changes, family interactions, other patient interactions, and the interactions of the helping professions. Thus the convalescent course of the patient following a dilatation and curettage (without complications) will be different from that of the patient who has had an uncomplicated convalescence after a hysterectomy. One or more of the convalescent phases will be extended or accentuated when a radical operation is necessary, when postoperative complications occur, when the patient is unable to or does not want to participate in her convalescence because of a physical or psychologic disequilibrium that seems overwhelming, or when disequilibrium is ignored, tolerated, or even accentuated by nonactivity or specific activity of the "helping" professions.

Period of survival mechanisms (injury phase)

The patient who has had anesthesia and surgical trauma must be able to utilize optimum protective and adaptive mechanisms for survival.

The total time span of this period for the patient with a major gynecologic operation extends from the immediate postanesthesia period to one or two days postoperatively. The period is one of shifting equilibrium in response to the stress of the anesthesia and to the injury or trauma of the operation.

Hospital administration divides this period into recovery room care and clinical unit care. Although seen in greater intensity in the recovery room, the same adaptive mechanisms continue during the entire one- to two-day postoperative period or the period of survival mechanisms. There are administrative advantages to a concentration of personnel and equipment for the postanesthesia patient when

---

*Moore, Francis D.: Metabolic care of the surgical patient, Philadelphia, 1959, W. B. Saunders Co., pp. 28-48.

close observation is necessary. The patient is then returned to the clinical unit after the time when close observation is no longer so necessary. There is also a disadvantage to this administrative division. Continuity of nursing is lost when a patient is moved from a preoperative unit to the surgical suite, to the recovery room, and back to the preoperative clinical unit. The "unknown" patient is "cared for" by many unknown and different nurses throughout a crucial period of time in her life. Even though the patient is exposed to many different experiences in each hospital area, there may be little or no communication from one unit to another about the patient, other than formal orders. As a result, each new nurse perceives this patient with little benefit of previous nursing knowledge and little awareness of the beneficial or detrimental influences accrued by the patient before she comes to the new unit. Titchener has emphasized the importance of such knowledge. "The quality and intensity of the emotional problems stirred by the onset of an illness, by the anticipation of surgical treatment, by the actual operation, or by the vicissitudes of the recovery and convalescence nearly always have consequences for the course of surgical treatment, and simultaneously they have effects upon subsequent psychological adjustment."* An awareness and an interpretation of each patient within each experience are necessary for extending the greatest help to the patient during her convalescence.

The postanesthesia patient

Even at the beginning of anesthesia, mechanisms in response to stress gain momentum. They are still present postanesthesia. There are two such mechanisms. (1) The sympathetic nervous system and the adrenal medulla are stimulated by emotion and surgical trauma. This mechanism is recognized as the "alarm" or the "fight or flight" syndrome described by Selye. (2) The other mechanism is the adrenal-cortical mechanism, stimulated by way of the sympathetic nervous system to the pituitary, which secretes ACTH and activates adrenocortical hormones. It is necessary to recognize and understand the immediate and expected adaptations that occur after any operation and anesthesia in order to protect the unconscious patient until later compensatory mechanisms take over. The immediate adaptive physical measures are in response to stress, the trauma of a wound, and fluid loss.

The *adrenal-cortical* response exerts two main adaptive influences. Hydrocortisone is concerned with the mobilization of food stores for increased metabolic needs. Aldosterone is concerned with the conservation of water and sodium during this crucial period of adjustment. Further discussion of clinical manifestations in relation to the cortical steroids will be found within later sections of the chapter.

The *sympathetic nervous system* response results in increased activity and therefore increased metabolism of vital organs. This includes an increased blood pressure, increased circulation to skeletal muscle and the vital organs such as the

---

*Titchener, James L., and Levine, Maurice: Surgery as a human experience, New York, 1960, Oxford University Press, p. 3.

heart, brain, liver, and kidneys, increased blood glucose, and increased blood coagulability. The mechanism provides immediate energy as an emergency measure in response to physical or emotional stress. At the same time, there is conservation of energy from areas that are not vital to the emergency measures, such as the skin, stomach, and intestines. The patient responding to mass sympathetic nervous system stimulation may be observed to be pale, with cool moist skin, and increased pulse and blood pressure.

The postoperative patient during this time of sympathetic nervous system influence is usually still unconscious and has flaccid skeletal muscles. This means that even after arousal muscular support or coordination is poor. It also means that the epiglottis functions slowly. Thus the usual protective device against aspiration of fluid or food into the bronchi is sluggish or even absent. The movements of the gastrointestinal tract are slowed, but the pyloric and cardiac sphincters may be hyperactive. The possibility of emesis exists in an individual whose defense mechanisms against aspiration are inhibited and who cannot even position herself advantageously for a gravity flow of the material from her mouth. *The maintenance of an open airway is the most important help given this patient until she can consciously control this for herself.* It is necessary to position the patient to straighten the airway and to remove those physical impediments that may occlude the airway, such as emesis, mucus in the mouth, or a relaxed tongue that may fall back and occlude the airway. During this period a gastric tube may be necessary.

Interpretation of vital signs. Tissue injury, blood loss, and pain are stressors that increase the production of epinephrine and norepinephrine and sympathetic nervous system effects. Clinical signs signal the presence or increase of these stressors within the postoperative period. When postoperative bleeding is present, a rising diastolic blood pressure (vasoconstriction due to the increasing production of norepinephrine) in the presence of a rapid pulse (increased epinephrine and norepinephrine) are early clinical warnings. A falling systolic blood pressure is a late sign of bleeding, indicating that adaptive and compensatory mechanisms have failed.

In order to make sound judgments about vital signs the nurse needs to know the preoperative level of the vital signs, the type and plane of the anesthetics used, and whether fluid or blood transfusion has been administered. For example, unless blood, packed cells, or a volume expander such as dextran is administered after blood loss, a lower blood pressure may be expected regardless of the fact that the patient may be receiving fluid replacement intravenously. While the fluid volume may be restored, the fluid viscosity remains lower than normal and the blood pressure remains lower.

It will be important for the nurse to know when certain anesthetics have been given. For example, cyclopropane or Fluothane may actually enhance bleeding by increasing peripheral vasodilatation and blood pressure. Other anesthetics administered in a deep plane may result in hypotension.

Obesity and age must also be considered in interpreting vital signs. The total blood volume varies inversely with obesity. There is less body water in the obese person than in the average person. There is also less total body water in a woman than in a man, since the body composition of the woman constitutes less muscle and more fat tissue. Therefore, a smaller loss of blood will produce more marked changes and earlier shock in the obese woman than in the average individual. It can also be anticipated that earlier and more severe trouble from fluid losses by emesis and gastric suction will occur in such an individual. In both the child and the elderly person the relationship of fluid volume to the total amount of body tissue is less than in the average adult. In both age extremes there is an intolerance to loss of fluid, resulting in rapid changes in blood pressure. Sclerosed vessels provide another variable to be considered as vital signs are evaluated in the elderly patient.

This elaboration of some observations and interpretations to be made from the blood pressure reading is not to mean that this interpretation is to be taken alone, but rather is to point out many of the factors involved in the interpretation of one vital sign. All vital signs are interrelated. The patient's temperature, pulse, respiration, and blood pressure are all considered in forming a judgment about the dynamic equilibrium of the patient at a particular moment in her postoperative course.

Immediate postoperative problems. Through constant vigilance and judgments by the nurse, postoperative problems can be recognized at the earliest possible time and immediate help can be summoned. This help may be from the gynecologist himself or from a consultant he has selected in another specialty such as general surgery, urology, or internal medicine.

Complications following gynecologic operations comprise those that may occur after any type of abdominal procedure as well as those peculiar to pelvic operation, both abdominal and vaginal. In the immediate postoperative period hypotensive shock, hemorrhage, aspiration, atelectasis, anuria, transfusion reaction, drug allergies, or acute gastric dilatation may occur.

Hemorrhage from the vagina may occur immediately or within several days following either abdominal or vaginal procedures. Even though the uterus may remain in situ, it cannot be assumed that vaginal bleeding is menstruation, although it could possibly be. In both abdominal and vaginal hysterectomies, bleeding may occur vaginally. For these reasons, all bleeding should be reported quickly and a medical judgment made. The only effective measure of treatment of continued bleeding after complete hysterectomy involves a return of the patient to the operating room, where the vaginal cuff can be examined and the source of bleeding sutured.

Internal hemorrhage may occur immediately after anesthesia or within several days postoperatively. Hypotension, tachycardia, abdominal distention, and tenderness with rebound indicate intra-abdominal hemorrhage. It is imperative to the patient's safety that everyone caring for gynecologic patients is watchful for any indication of postoperative bleeding.

Postoperative shock in gynecologic patients is unusual. It may occur after procedures such as radical hysterectomy with lymph node dissection, radical vulvectomy, or any procedure performed to correct a hemorrhagic condition such as a ruptured ectopic pregnancy. Careful preoperative evaluation of the stress reserves of the elderly patient and *careful* fluid replacement can forestall complications of postoperative shock.

The manner in which postoperative therapy is administered or the actual disruption of therapy may result in postoperative problems. Applied to intravenous therapy, these complications involve subcutaneous tissue damage caused by a needle or intracatheter that is out of the vein, the dangerous thrombus of a "lost" intracatheter, or pulmonary edema resulting from excessive or too rapidly administered fluids or blood over a short period of time. To detect complications promptly, the nurse must observe and examine frequently all patients receiving intravenous therapy.

Many major gynecologic operative procedures involve tissues adjacent to the urinary bladder. This means that the pressure exerted by a filling or distended bladder on the operative site should be eliminated. A clamped, kinked, or occluded indwelling catheter or its associated drainage tubing is a threat to the patient's welfare. The sympathetic nervous system influence may initially stimulate the patient's urinary output, while the influence of increasing aldosterone production after operative tissue injury will inhibit the urinary output. The amount of blood loss, the amount and kind of intravenous fluids given during and after the operation, the rate of administration, and the blood pressure of the patient will influence the amount of urinary output within the immediate hours after operation. These are factors that the nurse considers as she observes and evaluates the patient's course.

In the absence of urinary output, operative trauma of the ureters should be suspected and reported immediately. Injury to the ureter is probably the most serious nonlethal risk of pelvic operation. Whereas overt ureteral injury is usually recognized and repaired at the time of the operation, it may go unrecognized until the early postoperative period. *Unilateral* ureteral injury is identified by severe flank pain, an abdominal mass, and fever. Radioisotope renograms demonstrate varying degrees of ureteral obstruction, and excretory urography will indicate where the injury has occurred.

The prevention and early recognition of unnecessary trauma and actual danger to the patient often depend on the skill and judgment of the nurse who, of all members of the healing professions, still spends the most time at the patient's bedside. In some hospitals she is the only one present to evaluate, formulate judgments, and regulate the therapeutic plan during the attending doctor's absence.

The patient's family. During the postanesthesia time when the patient may still be unconscious, the family may or may not be in contact with the patient. If they are not allowed to actually see the patient, these may be long trying hours added to the hours of operation. If they are allowed to see the patient in the recovery room or in the patient's own room immediately postanesthesia, the family requires interpretation of the patient's condition. They cannot be expected to be reassured to see the unconscious patient, even though they were aware she would be this way. They may never have seen her unresponsive, and the paleness of her skin and its coolness and moistness may be very disconcerting to them. The presence of "all the tubes" may be explained to them as well as any activity of nursing care involving the patient. The very atmosphere of a recovery room implies the tenaciousness of life. It is easy for a family to make wrong assumptions from those actions or procedures that seem routine and necessary to members of the healing professions. Stress narrows and distorts accurate perception of even familiar events. When the unfamiliar is viewed within a stressful situation, gross distortions and fear can arise quickly.

The family may be very concerned with the patient's groans and moans, equating this with severe agony. This may be interpreted to them as the strivings of the semiconscious patient to communicate. It is explained that partially conscious patients can hear voices and that selective conversation at the bedside is indicated.

A family during this experience may hear no more than the very anxious patient did in the doctor's office. Direct person-to-person communication helps the family member focus on what is being said by selecting words they can understand, using a volume loud enough to reduce distractions, enunciating clearly, and looking directly at them to hold their attention. The family's helplessness at this time is extreme. They frequently feel they are in the way. It is an uncomfortable feeling to *want* to help but not to know *how* to help. The nurse becomes their substitute. For this reason, the nurse's feeling for the patient conveyed through her actions reassures them more than words. The manner in which an injection is given or the smooth, rhythmical turning and lifting of the patient reassure and reinforce the family's earlier anticipations of postoperative care.

Since the confident or the distraught family eventually influences the patient, the nurse seeks to answer these questions: "What are the ways to help this particular family so they will not feel in the way?" "What are the ways to help them so they will not feel *apologetic* for their concern for the patient?" "How can their presence and their concern be made more acceptable to the busy clinical staff?" The nurse who is concerned for the "whole patient" cannot exclude the patient's family.

The postarousal patient

William Golding has written an intense account of the struggle of self-survival.

He stopped shouting and strained his eyes to see through the darkness but it lay right against his eyeballs. He put his hand before his eyes and saw nothing. Immediately the terror of blindness added itself to the terror of isolation and drowning. He began to make vague climbing motions in the water. "Help! Is there anybody there? Help!" . . . His head fell forward. . . . "Exercise." He began to tread water gently. . . . "Cold. Mustn't get too cold. . . ." He began to thresh with his hands and force his body round. . . . [Then] he lay slackly in his life belt, allowing the swell to do what it would. . . . He thought. The thoughts were laborious, disconnected but vital. "Presently it will be daylight. I must move from one point to another. Enough to see one move ahead. Presently it will be daylight. . . . I won't die. I won't die. Not me—precious!" He roused himself with a sudden surge of feeling that had nothing to do with the touch of the sea. . . . "Help, somebody—help!"*

The patient, as she emerges from anesthesia, sometimes has feelings of struggle, falling back, resting once more, receiving auditory or tactile stimuli, rousing once more, having laborious and disjointed thoughts which trail off, and then a summoning of strength which brings her to the surface, alive again. This is seemingly random activity, but it is really purposeful poststress activity. These are the adaptions and struggles to survive the trauma of the operation and the anesthesia that put her to sleep. The degree of struggle seems related to preoperative anxiousness and also to the type of anesthesia used.

After complete arousal the patient usually lies quietly, with the desire to be undisturbed and to sleep. It is during this period that the patient begins to show more stable blood pressure. The pulse is still rapid and the temperature elevated, but the skin color, warmth, and dryness are improved. The latter are indications of diminishing stress and decreasing influences of the sympathetic nervous system. The presence of fear, pain, nausea, and vomiting often accentuate or prolong the sympathetic nervous system influences. Nausea and vomiting influence pain perception and create greater anxiety. Similarly, pain and anxiety as stressors influence increasing nausea and vomiting. The nurse assumes early responsibility for evaluation of the patient's pain, anxiety, nausea or vomiting, and their interrelationships and for the decision concerning her nursing activity.

Often what the patient most needs to receive is confidence in those who watch and minister to her so that she can sleep in a feeling of safety. She is very dependent during this period and willing to be so *if* she can trust those about her. In times of emergency and stress when energies are being conserved for vital tasks of survival, nonverbal communication becomes the language preference. Verbal communication is minimized and actually may be misunderstood. This is particularly true if the verbal content of communication is "You're fine, don't worry" and the nonverbal content is "I'm afraid," "I'm not sure in this situation," or "I wish she'd let me go; I'm late with my medications." When there is any conflict of meaning between verbal and nonverbal communication, the recipient disregards the weaker or the least reliable (to her) form. During times of stress, interpreted nonverbal content tends to be accepted by a patient and accompanying verbal content rejected if it conflicts. Conflicts and incongruence in communication systems arouse distrust toward the sender and anxiety about the interpreted message. They create future breaks in communication. As a direct result, the patient becomes depressed.

Specific responses of the patient. Specific responses of the patient involve the effects of movement on the wound, antidiuretic activity, mobilization of food stores, time distortion, and family interaction.

The wound and movement. Movement and stress on the wound are painful to

---

*Golding, William: Pincher Martin, New York, 1956, Capricorn Books, pp. 11-13.

the patient after arousal. Sudden thoughtless movement initiated by her will hurt and she will be reluctant to attempt movement again. Postoperative patients often lie rigid, fearing even more pain if they try to move from an already uncomfortable position. The nurse may help the patient most advantageously by evaluating her position and state of comfort and then by helping her to turn or move in the most painless ways. Careful and assisted turning of the conscious patient for the first time prepares her to accomplish later turning by herself, with diminishing degrees of tension, anxiety, and pain. In assisting the patient by those means that produce the least amount of stress on the abdominal incision, the patient may be reminded to put one leg over the other, to put the arm over the chest in the same direction, and to roll easily. By helping, encouraging, and using the same routine each time, the patient can begin to participate. As the family repeatedly observes the same routine, they too can begin to assist. They thereby help the patient and relieve their own tension. The best way for *this* patient, the easiest way, and the preferred side are worked out between the nurse and the patient. This is the kind of information that should be reported from one change of nurses to another in order to have nursing continuity for the individual patient.

Because stasis in blood vessels may lead to postoperative phlebitis, the patient is encouraged and reminded to move her legs frequently. Movement of her legs up and down, that is, sliding on the flat of her feet, is more comfortable than to slide her legs sideways with her legs flat on the bed. Legs flexed at the knees relieve the tension and contraction of the abdominal sheath, and since this is a comfortable experience to the patient, she may request a pillow or gatch under her knees. However, pressure on the popliteal vessels may further increase the possibility of stasis in the lower extremities. With no support under her knees, the patient will freely move her legs up and down as comfort dictates. Thereby, two functions are performed in one patient activity: comfort and prevention of stasis.

Antidiuretic activity. One of the early adaptive processes in the postoperative patient is an increased production of aldosterone. Aldosterone acts directly on the kidney tubules and influences the retention of water, sodium, and chloride in response to fluid losses. Therefore, unless much intravenous fluid has been given, little urinary output is expected or possible within a 24-hour period after operation. The total output during this time is usually limited to 450 to 1,000 ml. This factor should be taken into account in the nurse's evaluation of the postoperative urinary output and in her evaluation of the time expected for the patient to void. Pressure of a distended bladder may cause pain in the operative site. It can also be detrimental to the operated area. Thus postoperative observation of the gynecologic patient must be more concerned with the time and amounts of voided urine than for other patients. Continuous drainage of the bladder by indwelling catheter or repeated catheterizations control the initial retention and later residual retention of urine.

MANAGEMENT OF URETHRAL CATHETERIZATION. During the past several years a controversy has been raging in medical literature regarding the use of intermittent urethral catheterization versus continuous bladder drainage for gynecologic patients. The bacteriologic problems of the urethral catheter have received the greatest attention. Complications from the use of the urethral catheter result when this instrument is used more frequently than required, when it is used without strict aseptic technique, and when it is withheld when specifically indicated.

A "clean" voided midstream collected specimen obtained after cleansing the urethra and a small pledget of cotton placed in the vagina should, in most instances, be adequate for microscopic examination. Catheterization need not be avoided if a sterile urine sample is necessary for the diagnosis of infection.

When the urinary tract requires drainage, failure to provide it can jeopardize the health of the patient. In like manner, indiscriminate use of the catheter is condemned. The postoperative patient should be given every opportunity and assistance to void normally. If she is unable, drainage of the bladder is indicated. Whether intermittent catheterization or continuous bladder drainage is the chosen method, adherence to the proper uses of the catheter is essential. These are strict surgical asepsis, including sterilization of the catheter, preparation of the urethra, a well-lubricated catheter of the appropriate size, and the insertion of the catheter; gentle manipulation of the catheter to prevent trauma to the mucous membrane; and aseptic management of the drainage equipment if constant drainage is utilized. The three most common sites of contamination in the continuous drainage setup are at the junction of the catheter and urethra, the point connecting the catheter to the drainage tubing, and the end of the tube in the collecting container. Contamination most frequently occurs when aseptic technique is not observed as the collecting container is emptied or when the clamped catheter is disconnected from the drainage tubing for the ambulating patient. Infection should be rare when continuous drainage of the bladder or intermittent catheterization is performed with careful aseptic technique.

Catheterization should be performed with a thorough knowledge of the anatomy and a concern for the patient who is experiencing embarrassment with the procedure. This means preparation of the patient prior to the catheterization and a concern for her protection from unnecessary exposure and the possibility of someone coming into the room while the procedure is being performed. Throughout, the manual deftness and confidence of the nurse determine the degree of muscle relaxation and confidence in the patient.

Because of possible distortions in the perineal area due to the operative procedure itself, the presence of sutures, or edema, the choice of small catheters in good condition is imperative after gynecologic operative procedures. Difficulty to pass a catheter beyond the meatus is usually due to the constriction of a sphincter in the middle third of the urethra or about ½ inch beyond the meatus. This sphincter, composed of striated muscle tissue, contracts whenever fear, anxiety, or pain are present. This indicates that the patient in pain should be given analgesia *before* catheterization is attempted. (The relief of pain also often permits spontaneous voiding.) The importance of the nurse-patient relationship in minimizing fear and anxiety prior to and during the catheterization is also emphasized. When sphincter constriction *is* encountered, a short hestitation of the catheter tip at this point (which provides a sustained stimulation of the muscle fiber) will fatigue the sphincter muscle. As the muscle relaxes, the catheter can be slowly and *easily* extended into the bladder. Talking to the patient as the catheter is inserted and requesting her to bear down (thus utilizing an antagonistic muscle group) will also reduce the transient difficulties sometimes encountered in catheterization of women.

The nurse may have her own feelings about the catheterization procedures, which in turn are interpreted in some way by the patient. The nurse may dislike the procedures. If she ignores the indwelling catheter except to periodically empty the collection container, she may imply neglect to the patient. If she exposes the patient, she implies insensitivity and unconcern for the patient's feelings. If she considers the catheterization schedule time consuming or the procedure itself difficult, the patient may feel humiliated and even experience a feeling of being responsible for the time expenditure or for creating a distasteful procedure for the nursing personnel. The patient who requires repeated catheterization may feel embarrassed every time the procedure must be accomplished. On the other hand, the patient who has an indwelling catheter often feels as though she is "tied to the bed." She cannot move freely without being aware of the tubing and the "gentle" tug that reminds her to turn over slowly, even when she is about to do this in her sleep. At no time is she more aware of being tied to her tubing or collecting container than when she gets out of bed for the first few times and, of necessity, must struggle as she walks along to make sure that the tubing does not get in her way and that the bag or bottle does not fall.

American citizens, with private bathrooms and modern plumbing, are very discreet about excreta. However, as soon as the patient is admitted to an American hospital, she is expected to speak freely about her excreta to strangers, albeit professional personnel, and sometimes even in the presence of her visitors. She is expected to assume a sense of equanimity and even observational skill toward her own excreta and other patients' within the room. The personnel of the hospital assume that this has no effect on patients. Would a urinary drainage bottle or bag be without effect to the adolescent patient expecting a visit from her peers? Would it be without effect to any other hospitalized woman who receives her visitors in her hospital room as a social event? The patient is often placed in situations that are sources of varying degrees of embarrassment or humiliation. These produce physiologic and psychologic responses. If these occasions are intense or numerous, or if they occur at periods when the patient is physically weak and vulnerable, the patient's response of defensiveness, withdrawal, or depression may be unduly prolonged and seemingly out of proportion to the triggering situation. It may have a sweeping or cumulative effect that arouses latent feelings concerning the operation, other troubling hospital incidents, or family concerns.

Mobilization of food stores. As a result of sympathetic nervous system activity after operation, the tone of the entire gastrointestinal tract is reduced. Even in the absence of nausea or vomiting, the patient usually has little interest in food during this period. In addition, it is usual that the intake of food and fluids by mouth is medically restricted until the sympathetic nervous system influences diminish. Overloading of the gastrointestinal tract before peristalsis resumes and before sphincter tone returns to normal results in gastrointestinal cramping and pain, not to be minimized by anyone who has ever felt it.

Until the patient can tolerate food, she is dependent on body food reserves. Metabolism continues and may be higher than usual due to the increased demands of the surgical wound and an elevated temperature, which may remain elevated until the end of the period of survival mechanisms (one to two days). During the entire postoperative period the wound has priority for food requirements. To accommodate the demand, reserves of body food are mobilized. This is another adaptive mechanism initiated for survival and one that is continued throughout the later periods of the convalescence to achieve optimum wound healing.

SOURCES OF FOOD AND WATER STORES. Muscle and liver glycogen are utilized immediately poststress (the anesthesia and operation) during the period of greatest sympathetic nervous influences. (It may be remembered that blood sugar is elevated due to this influence.) The sources of this immediate food are usually exhausted within 8 to 16 hours. This means that other sources of body food must be tapped.

Body *fat* is a main source of reserve food. After the trauma of a major operation, 250 to 500 grams or 2,000 to 4,500 calories per day may be obtained from body fat. Since women are more heavily endowed with body fat than men, there is usually no problem with this available source of food for the gynecologic patient. Children, adolescents, the elderly, and cachectic patients usually have little fat.

The breakdown of *muscle* provides another source of food for the patient. As muscle tissue diminishes, nitrogen and potassium are lost from the cells. During this period the patient is considered to be in *negative* nitrogen balance. This is the period of catabolism. There is more tissue destruction than tissue rebuilding. Tissue has not only been destroyed due to the injury of the operation, but muscle tissue is being destroyed or broken down for food needs.

As these tissues are being utilized as sources of food, new sources of water become available to the patient. Therefore, if the patient receives no intravenous fluids in the postoperative period, the adaptive processes not only conserve or retain water by changing the kidney tubule absorption threshold but also provide a new source of water through the oxidation of fat and the lysis of muscle tissue. Oxidation of 0.5 kilogram (1 pound) of fat produces 500 ml. of water; the lysis of 1 kilogram (2.2 pounds) of muscle tissue produces 250 ml. of water. The obese individual has less total water volume per body mass and cannot tolerate sudden water demands or fluid losses. However, if these changes are slow enough and extend over a period of time, she has quantities of water available as her own fat is oxidized. Obesity, old age, youth, the presence of fever, an extensive wound, blood loss, diaphoresis, an increased respiratory rate, or any other increased metabolic demand increases the need for more body water in the postoperative patient.

The availability of these food and water reserves by the patient should be understood by the nurse. There are specific patients who can be reassured with a simplified accounting of these mechanisms. Many nationalities place high value on the positive relationships between food and health. Such individuals have a tendency to urge rapid food intake in the postoperative period. They tend to equate the rate of convalescence with the amount of food taken and the promptness with which eating is begun. If these patients and families were cognizant of the adaptive mechanisms that supply energy to the patient before oral food can be tolerated, they would perhaps be less apprehensive and less fearful. Patients and families do not ordinarily appreciate the caloric value within the bottles of water-appearing intravenous fluids. They usually are assured of the patient's nutrition only when oral feeding is possible.

Time distortion. During this time and in varying degrees during the entire period of the survival mechanisms, the patient experiences an element of time distortion. There are timeless periods when hours merge, and daylight and night are the only measures of time. In the presence of an elevated body temperature, minutes are (subjectively) shorter than normal. Therefore, an actual clock hour to a patient seems longer than her experienced hour. Observation of patients seems to indicate that increased time distortion also occurs in the presence of pain and anxiety. When the patient looks back on this period of her postoperative course, she remembers only fragments of an indescribably long span of time. They are her "lost days."

Patient and family interaction. During most of this period there is a general disinterest by the patient in her surroundings, in all instructions and urgings by medical personnel, and also in her visitors. The first day she may frequently check to see whether the family is close at hand. Otherwise she seldom makes an effort to communicate with them, feeling satisfied that only their presence is necessary. Occasionally, the family may feel shut out. Their concern for the patient remains high, and they may respond subjectively to the patient's pain, nausea, or restlessness. The family often has to assume that all is going well in this period by the absence of commotion or by the lack of any emergency measures. The nurse is frequently in and out of the room, and this does provide them with reassurance. However, families observe that nurses go in and out of a room, check on equipment, or observe the patient, but they do not speak to them or even look at them.

The family needs to know what is going on. Optimum nurse-doctor relationships are essential if the nurse is to know what has been done, what has been told to the family, how they have understood this, and what she may now tell them to reassure and help them. Care of "only" the patient is not enough. The anxious, distraught family, often banished to the hall, has a very real effect on the patient, who readily picks up nonverbal communications from them. She is affected by interpersonal stressor elements. She may interpret her family's responses as indications of the precariousness of her own situation, of her family's distrust of those on whom she is dependent, or of her family's anger or hurt suffered from someone from whom she must ask help.

If patients sometimes are silent and do not ask for help when they experience pain, unusual postoperative feelings, or mounting fears, it may be because the "helping" professions have not made it easy for the patient to accept that help. If patients sometimes *demand* instant action or continuous activity from the professions, it may be because these patients feel precarious in their situation. They cannot afford to be submissive and ask. There is always the risk that a request may be denied or ignored. It may be that the experiences of the family may anger or depress the patient to the extent that she will squander postoperative energy resources in detrimental or unhappy interpersonal relationships. During this period wide fluctuations of metabolic and endocrine function may occur in response to interpersonal incidents in which the patient feels hopeless or depressed or in which the patient feels directly or indirectly threatened, with no means of coping with the situation. Interpersonal relationships with the professions, other hospital personnel, the family, or roommates can be stressors and, therefore, deterrents to the healing process. They can also provide beneficial adjuncts to the therapy and the healing process.

Later responses of the patient. Later responses of the patient concern her experiences on the first postoperative night and ambulation.

First postoperative night. The success of the first postoperative night is dependent on many factors. Can the patient be assured that everything is under control? Can she trust her safety? Can she afford to go to sleep? How well does she know the personnel who are on in the evenings? How has she gotten along with the personnel during the day? Has she felt that she has been in control in any way? Has she been a partner or a participant in some small measure in her own "recovery"? What does she know or dread of the next day?

As the evening personnel prepare the patient for sleep, many of these questions will be answered for her. Not all of them will be answered verbally. She will find the answers in many of the ways in which they move her and communicate in other nonverbal ways. Fresh linen or newly adjusted linen, a correctly placed and "just right" pillow, a change in position, and other small rituals of preparation for sleep indicate to the patient the concern of others. Comfort measures and confidence prior to receiving an analgesic will enhance the activity of the analgesic. Comfort, trust, an analgesic, and a sedative may guarantee the patient a restful and sleep-filled postoperative night.

Ambulation. The patient is urged to ambulate at a time of diminishing food reserves and therefore at a time when increasing energy conservation exists. She is urged to ambulate at a time of diminishing muscle mass and therefore decreasing muscle strength. This is not to negate the importance of early ambulation to the patient in terms of a reduction of complications, a restoration of circulation in the extremities, a reduction of muscle rigidity, a reduction of pain in the wound, and an actual preservation of muscle mass by muscle use. It *is* to emphasize that mobilization counters the free use of muscle by the body as a food reserve and that mobilization increases the metabolic requirements of the individual as a result of the activity.

This has significant implications for nursing. The time of ambulation, its extent, and its duration are judgments that are made individually for each patient by each nurse for each ambulation during the postoperative period. For example, the elderly patient, because of age, has a smaller and weaker muscle mass due to collagen changes; because of her sex, she has a lower proportion of muscle tissue to body weight than a man. Wasting of muscle postoperatively leaves the elderly patient an even smaller muscle mass than usual. Therefore, muscle weakness and lack of strength can be anticipated in many aged patients, leaving little power available for their ambulation. Arthritic skeletal changes, the effects of stress, and possible changes in body coordination imply still other modifications in the ambulation of the aged person.

Early ambulation of *any* patient is an important nursing activity. Adequate assistance for support of the wound and the patient are essentials. Equally important is the accurate interpretation of those developing signs peculiar to each patient which indicate that the patient is becoming tired. To be "tired" is used in this connotation as a gradual losing of strength and energy due to exertion. The patient returned to bed after showing unique signs of growing tired (which will probably be entirely nonverbal cues) will usually state her regret that she could not please the nurse by staying up longer and fulfilling the "to the minute" requirement. To herself, she will admit surprise and, after a short rest, will feel the exhilaration of her physical achievement. She will be encouraged that the wound is still intact (one of the unstated worries of all early ambulated patients) and that pain was not increased. The patient will be willing and anxious to get up again. She has achieved something; she is better than she thought possible. Her family will be encouraged and happy. To this patient the act of early mobilization has a beneficial effect on her convalescence in many ways.

"Fatigue" and "exhaustion" may be equated equally. The fatigued or exhausted patient is completely spent with exertion. Her physical and emotional reserves are depleted, and the most neglected patient allowed to become fatigued will exhibit signs of sympathetic nervous system responses to stress: emotional lability, perspiration, skin paleness, rapid pulse, changes in blood pressure, faintness, and a resumption of experienced nausea, emesis and/or pain. The *fatigued* patient has received no benefit from the ambulation. Physiologically and emotionally, she actually has been retarded in her convalescence. Depending on the level of fatigue or exhaustion experienced and the extent of the depletion of her physical and emotional reserves, the patient may revert to the immediate postoperative stress period. As she is returned to bed, she will further insulate herself from all immediate demands upon her. She has felt no achievement in getting up. She indeed may lie rigidly and move less than before the experience. To the patient the experience has substantiated the fact that she *is* very weak and helpless. Her sense of helplessness, dependency on others, and their failure to help her may be experienced as hopelessness and despondency. Such events have detrimental effects on restorative processes and on an already prevailing negative nitrogen balance. Her immediate defeat will have an effect on future ambulation periods and will have possible future influences on her entire convalescence and wound healing. Well-intentioned medical management for the patient during the period of survival mechanisms can be nonbeneficial or detrimental to the patient when *nursing* is not extended to the patient.

Period of restorative mechanisms

The patient must be able to utilize optimum restorative mechanisms for wound healing and to prepare for the resumption of her role within the home.

The stress period for the patient has passed. She now enters periods of increasing stability. Biologically, these are focused on the healing of the wound and general physical rehabilitation; psychologically, these periods are focused on "healing" the wound of a missing organ, of an interrupted function or a changed appearance, and on self-rehabilitation; socially, these periods are focused on a restoration of the patient and family within a family unit and friendship group, which may be the same as before the hospitalization or which may now contain new or adjusted functions.

The patient now begins to show increasing interest in her surroundings. For the patient with major gynecologic surgery this occurs about the second or third day postoperative. Time becomes punctuated by meal times, periodic procedures, and visits from family, friends, and medical staff. The patient shows interest in the visit of her family and doctor. She begins to anticipate the visit, to know its approximate clock time, and "to plan" so that nursing activities will be completed *before* the time of the visit. The doctor's visit becomes a professional call *and* a social event.

The patient makes this transition seemingly "all at once." One day she is still down under and the next (usually the second or third postoperative day) she greets her doctor and family with, "I feel fine today." Actually, this has been a gradually changing sequence of diminishing stress factors to an increasing state of stability and equilibrium. She is now able to tolerate food and to enjoy it, she is afebrile, and even with moderate ambulation her vital signs are stable. Her urinary output has increased and approaches a normal balance with her fluid intake.

Her bursts of physical, emotional, and intellectual activity exceed her energy reserves, which have not been restored and are still low. As a result, at the beginning of the period of restoration, her bursts of energy are quickly dissipated. Her initial eagerness in participating in her own morning care often ends in disappointment in herself and frustration in her weakness; her predetermined goal to walk as far as the nursing station may be unfulfilled, and her progress may not seem as positive to her as five minutes before; her enthusiasm and joy in receiving visitors may dim as the demands of being hostess to her guests deplete her energy. She may buoyantly greet her doctor one minute and dissolve in the "weeps" the next. Emotional release and sudden onset of physical weakness are *usual* at this stage of convalescence. Its presence is discouraging to the patient, frightening to her family or friends, and often misunderstood or impatiently tolerated by the nursing staff. The patient should be prepared for and reassured about the fluctuating nature of this stage and encouraged to recognize early signs of tiring. She can also be protected from her own overambitious plans of self-care, ambulation, and social roles. This means that the patient and the nurse together set realistic and yet flexible goals of activity for the day and for the hour. It also means that the nurse helps relieve the patient of these activities *before* they are physically excessive and *before* the patient experiences disappointment in herself and in her progress. One very perceptive student told her instructor, "I arranged her unit as comfortably and conveniently for her as I could. Then I helped her to feel no shame when she had to return to rest."

Specific responses of the patient. Specific responses of the patient during the restorative period are wound and food demands, gastrointestinal activity, social outturning, and self-rehabilitation.

The wound and food demands. The increased activity of the patient is possible because of a decreasing experience of pain in the wound with movement. Increased movement also seems to decrease the wound discomfort. This is true of patients with vaginal incisions as well as those with abdominal incisions. Warm perineal cleansing or external douching decreases discomfort of the perineal incision. In the presence of optimum healing, the wound is clean and dry and gradually loses the red color of its incised edges as granulation accelerates. Tingling, pulling, tugging, or twinges are described by patients in their later pain experiences with the wound. Removal of sutures about the fifth to seventh day usually affords the patient some relief of these sensations. Without the sutures, however, she usually requires reassurances of the tensile strength of the incision.

This is the period of anabolism or tissue rebuilding, when the wound must acquire strength exclusive of the surgical sutures. The wound still has priority for all food. Therefore, as the activity of the patient increases and her body food reserves steadily decrease, it is imperative that her oral food intake increases.

The patient's appetite returns during this period, though in the beginning a full meal may be abandoned after a little is eaten. When the nurse is aware of the capricious appetite of the patient, she can enhance the patient's continued interest in food by appraising the tray of food *before* the patient receives it. When the appearance of the tray itself and the main plate are esthetically pleasing, when the portions of food are moderate or even small, and when the hot foods are hot and the cold foods really cold, the patient usually becomes surprised that she enjoys food once more. Thoughtful dietary planning for the early convalescent patient also involves in-between meals and before-bedtime snacks. This assures a more constant food intake at a time when energy demands are high and when tissue rebuilding (the wound and depleted body food stores) is imperative. Later, sufficient quality and quantity can be accomplished in three conventional meals.

Initiative in the guidance and wise selection of food during this period should be undertaken by the nurse and dietitian with the patient. Fruit plates and desserts offer color and appetite appeal to the patient. This is, of course, necessary to stimulate and sustain a wavering appetite. However, these foods afford her no protein intake. Patients given the opportunity to select their own food require postoperative guidance for the food choices most advantageous for their physical restoration. These patients need to know that depleted protein food reserves now require replacement and that wound healing is dependent on sufficient intake of protein and vitamin C foods. Water intake, too, should be encouraged.

Gastrointestinal activity. As the normal function of the stomach is restored, bowel activity returns. A few patients may accomplish the first postoperative elimination without enemas about the third or fourth postoperative day. Enemas will be necessary for most patients and will make this initial elimination less painful stress on the wound.

Social outturning of the patient. As the patient becomes stronger, she becomes increasingly interested in those about her: her roommate, patients down the hall, the nurses, and of course her family. Environmental effects of the hospital and of its staff on the patient and her convalescence have been enumerated. The environmental effects of other roommates on the patient, friends, family, and her own home on the patient's convalescence cannot be ignored. They give her encouragement and motivation for rapid restoration. They can also give her time pressures and worries when small children are in the care of others, when the husband alone is holding the family together, and when financial obligations mount.

Patient worry often occurs after visiting hours. Unrecognized and unaided, the patient with uncertain energy may show physical symptoms of sleeplessness, an elevated temperature, increased pulse, greater fatigue, and early signs of returned stress. Patient problems big enough to enter the hospital with her also become the problems of the helping-healing professions. Early referral to the profession best able to help, such as social workers or hospital chaplains, is often essential for the patient's welfare. Referral to other professions concerned with the patient in no way minimizes the responsibilities of the doctor-nurse relationship. Rather, it increases that responsibility. Every individual concerned with the patient during her hospitalization increases the complexity of the patient's relationships. The level of the doctor-nurse relationship determines how these interactions can be coordinated and generally interpreted to the patient and her family.

Self-rehabilitation. As the patient is helped to increasing degrees of physical activity, she also requires time and help to handle the psychologic processes of her restoration as a woman, wife, and mother. After the initial period of postoperative stress or after the patient's fight to survive, she can be assailed by self-questioning: "Why did this happen to me?" The patient who has had a hysterectomy may now be completely confronted with the reality and finality of the operative procedure. She can no longer minimize the operation. If her denial of the illness and the extent of the operation has been excessive, she may be suddenly overwhelmed by the realization that the past cannot be restored. She grieves for her loss and for the past. To the helping professions this means that she needs understanding, concern of others, and time in order to be able to consider the past, adjust to the present, and eventually plan a future. As members of a helping-healing profession, nurses are uniquely available to the patient at times when these thoughts are uppermost. As the nurse is the same sex, the patient can identify with her; the nurse can communicate with the patient *if* she knows herself and her own fears. The nurse can help the husband or family during this time as she accepts and interprets the patient's feelings for them.

If the patient has no time for these thoughts and feelings because of many visitors, constant television distraction, or the diverting tactics of friends and even nurses from "morbid" thoughts, she may go home unprepared and have to work out this adjustment alone. Her ability and willingness to recognize, explore, and try herself as a "new or different" person should begin in the hospital with the help of the helping professions. Crying is an emotional release. It should not be inhibited or feared when the postoperative patient cries. Its presence indicates that the power of the situation is recognized and that the patient is submissive. Crying indicates that the patient needs to be sustained until she has the time and energy to adjust or cope with her changed situation.

The patient takes a new inventory of herself and of herself with her family as they visit her within the hospital. Her restructuring proceeds as she interprets evidences of a secure and loved relationship with them. When this work of convalescence is accompanied by increasing physical activity and strength, the patient seeks to go home. If the patient's marital relationship has been precarious prior to operation, the absence of evidences of love and concern for her during the convalescent period may delay the patient's ability to resolve her grief. The loss of a reproductive organ may be accorded excessive and prolonged importance. Counsel should be sought for such patients early.

Restoration period problems. The physical problems that accrue during this period are inherent in changing gastrointestinal function and demand, changing wound integrity, diminished globulin, and increased activity. They have been discussed in detail at the beginning of the chapter.

Home preparations. An evaluation of the patient's readiness to go home should be made by all members of the healing professions in contact with her. This means the presence of good wound healing, increasing physical stamina, degree of the patient's participation in her convalescence, and expressed or unexpressed desire of the patient to resume her family role.

The nurse helps the patient and family anticipate and therefore prevent some problems involved in the patient's return home. Identified while the patient is still in the hospital, the solutions may often be worked out before the patient's discharge. For some of these, the services of social workers may be indicated. Other problems may easily be taken care of by the family *when* they are aware of them. Some of these might be as follows: Will the patient be able to walk up two or three flights of stairs to an apartment or to a bedroom in a bilevel home? If not, certain arrangements will have to be made before discharge. The patient who has had minor or major surgery will be unable to assume the full mantle of responsibility as soon as she arrives home, even though members of the family may feel she should and may feel relieved to have things back to normal. Who will share her responsibilities with her? How will the children greet the patient? How should the children be prepared before the patient's discharge? How does a mother or a grandmother after operation resist the upturned arms of the small child asking to be *lifted* and held? If the question is raised and the solution suggested *before* the patient is faced with this dilemma, the patient and a happy child will be helped. If there will be dressings to be changed, can the patient do this and does she know where to obtain more? Does she know how long to expect a discharge to continue, when she can expect a resumption of her menses, and what new bleeding in the patient with a hysterectomy might mean after being home about a month? Such anticipations of the patient's adjustments in the home are nursing responsibilities. They are followed up by realistic problem solving with the patient and family and the special assistance of the doctor. Only when concern exists for those factors that influence the patient's welfare in and out of the hospital can it be modestly said that the welfare and worth of the "whole" individual are respected and "cared" for.

RECOMMENDED READINGS FOR STUDENTS

Kaufman, M. Ralph, et al.: The emotional impact of ward rounds, New York State Journal of Medicine 57:3193-3205, 1957.

Ruesch, Jurgen, and Kees, Weldon: Non-verbal communication: Notes on the visual perception of human relations, Berkeley, 1964, University of California Press, Chapters 2 and 3.

RECOMMENDED READINGS FOR INSTRUCTORS

Beecham, C. T., editor: Complications of gynecologic surgery, Clinical Obstetrics and Gynecology 5:499-596, 1962.

Desautels, Robert E., and Harrison, J. Hartwell: The mismanagement of the urethral catheter, Medical Clinics of North America 43:1573-1584, 1959.

Gerbie, A. B., and Flanagan, C. L.: Gynecologic applications of the radioisotope renogram, American Journal of Obstetrics and Gynecology 84:1838, 1962.

Moore, Francis D.: Metabolic care of the surgical patient, Philadelphia, 1959, W. B. Saunders Co., pp. 28-48.

Titchener, James L., and Levine, Maurice: Surgery as a human experience, New York, 1960, Oxford University Press, pp. 192-203.

Chapter 5

The adolescent patient

Adolescence is recognized as a time of change and transition. Obvious physical changes occur, transforming the girl into a woman. A girl becomes very conscious of her body and bodily processes. It is a period of wide emotional ranges, when idealism runs high and disappointment and disillusionment are frequent. It is a time when everything is either white or black, when facts require proof, and yet gross generalizations are easily made on the strength of the peer group. Freedom from elder authority is demanded, but peer authority is asked for and readily accepted despite its usual rigidity. Parental authority is often ignored, while adult models are actively mimicked.

Care of the adolescent girl by the young student nurse is frequently difficult. If it is considered that the social and psychologic period of female adolescence extends to ages 18 to 21 years, it can be appreciated that many student nurses find themselves in the awkward position of being an authoritative figure to their peers. They may be uncomfortably like the patient.

Understanding a patient begins with self-understanding, with movement toward recognition and acceptance of similarities and differences in the other. This is more difficult when the other closely mirrors the nurse herself. The student nurse, however, has an advantage in her relationship with the adolescent patient: she does know how to speak her language. With optimum communication and with the guidance of a sensitive teacher, the difficulties of an adolescent–young nurse relationship can be surmounted.

THE NURSE AND THE ADOLESCENT

It is toward initial understanding of the adolescent girl as a gynecologic patient that this chapter has been developed. The influence of the nurse within nursing interactions or as a citizen, neighbor, or friend is to be emphasized. Within her role as a woman and through the sanctions of a helping profession, her importance is fourfold. These four are as follows:

1. To interpret to the adolescent and her parents the developmental changes and their effects on adolescent thought and behavior. A nurse is uniquely available to help and guide the adolescent through the fears and problems of this period. As a woman and a member of a helping profession she has potential abilities to strengthen the growth and understanding of the adolescent toward maturity. The sanctions of her profession make it possible for her to be both teacher and model. Within these roles she can interpret and mediate the two generations of adolescent and parent. Cultural influences and old wives' tales affect the adolescent girl and her future attitudes toward femininity, menstruation, marriage, childbearing, and menopause. The adolescent patient of today may be a different woman tomorrow because of the influences of the helping professions.

2. To recognize the unspoken fears and anticipate the unrecognized problems of the ill adolescent. Gynecologic fears and symptoms may coexist and complicate a primary and "unrelated" illness. Amenorrhea, spotting of blood, and early or late menses may be created by the anxieties and stresses of hospitalization and/or medical-surgical therapies, *or* by the ongoing life stresses of the adolescent-adult worlds. The early identity of these gynecologic problems and their manifestations in the adolescent often depend on the perceptive ability of the nurse and the quality of her patient-nurse relationship.

3. To teach interdependence and therefore the ability to give and receive. Adolescence is a denial of dependence and a demand for independence. Illness and hospitalization frustrate these important goals for the adolescent. Since nurses have the ability to enhance the hospital or clinic environment, they have the ability to provide conditions that allow the adolescent to maintain self-worth, autonomy, and growth. They can also provide the environment that makes it easier for the adolescent to seek and accept help. Dependence is not always a sign of immaturity nor independence a sure sign of maturity. Maturity may be measured by an individual's *inter*dependence with others or the ability to both give and receive. The student nurse and the adolescent patient can learn together to give and receive in such a relationship. Interdependence as an experienced concept can be one of the most important aspects of care to the adolescent and one of the most enduring and maturing benefits of that care. Thus the adolescent can learn to become responsible for her own health and to assume responsibility with the mutual help and trust of others.

4. To assist in fulfilling the optimum therapeutic regimen for the adolescent, recognizing throughout those unique fears of the adolescent as they relate to any physical awareness, illness, and differences from others.

What situations create the time and place when a nurse assumes the role of teacher and model to the adolescent? The potential responsibility exists whenever nurse and adolescent are together, whether the setting is a summer camp, a home, a doctor's office, a school, a clinic, or a hospital. Perhaps of all these locales, the nurses within the camp, school, and clinic are most cognizant of this responsibility. They have assumed teaching as a role that supplements and/or complements the family's teaching, and in some instances they have fully accepted the role of surrogate mother, especially in the camp or private school. For the hospitalized adolescent the nurse is also the surrogate mother during those periods when the natural mother is not at the bedside. Therefore, it is often the nurse's role to prepare the hospitalized preadolescent with a long-term chronic illness for the physical changes taking place. The usual sophistication of such patients with "hospital" terminology will necessitate a different "curriculum" for this student-patient than for the newly admitted acutely ill patient who begins to menstruate for the first time.

One measure of a good teacher is her ability to adapt the teaching material to the ability of the learner and her ability to measure the extent or intensity of the learner's present motivation or need for learning. Applied to the nurse and her adolescent patient, this means the following:

1. In the presence of a teacher-learner relationship she interprets the existing level of comprehension at *this immediate time* of the relationship. The individual adolescent will communicate and interpret previously learned material in a different manner and context today than she did yesterday or than she will tomorrow. The patient is different today in this present encounter with this particular nurse than she would be with another. It is this changing and dynamic character of people in their environment and with one another that necessitates the *art* of teaching and the *art* of nursing. It is this quality of teaching and nursing that defies static routines or lesson plans and demands individual sensitivity for experiencing, interpreting, and acting (teaching and/or nursing) within the living situation.

2. In the presence of a teacher-learner relationship she guides the introduction of new material, chooses the means of communication and devices of clarification (anecdotes, word pictures, analogies, etc.), and synthesizes this with previously known material, according to the cues, verbal and nonverbal, given by the adolescent patient.

3. Some of these cues may mean: "You're going too fast"; "I don't understand you, but you'll think I'm dumb if I tell you"; "I can't believe that, I won't believe that"; "That's wrong"; or "That's different than what I've learned before; who's right?" The interpretation of such cues influences not only the content level but also the optimum amount of content for the present situation.

4. Recognition and interpretation of such cues of verbal or nonverbal communication imply that both nurse and patient, teacher and learner, are in some measure effectively communicating and understanding one another. This is based on the knowledge that each individual has some effect on the other within any situation and that this influences and counterinfluences each individual's perception and response within each situation. Added to this are changing environmental or physical factors that influence the individuals during this particular situation.

Thus it is that no two student nurses can effectively nurse and teach a single patient in exactly the same way, use the same content, nor cover the same area of content, for the patient responds to each one differently and they to the patient at each single encounter. It is therefore not enough to know the why, how, and what of any subject content or the facts, rationale, and underlying principles. Anyone who teaches is sensitive to the effect her communication is having upon the learner; she is stimulated, bored, overwhelmed, or frightened by the message, or she accepts, rejects, or denies it. The teacher is also aware of the effect of the learner upon her. Her teaching relationship is uniquely influenced by the learner who is compliant, anxious, eager, or willing to please. It also is influenced by the learner who is resistant to her offers of help, asks probing questions, is not satisfied with the answers given, repeats the same questions, does not show evidences of learning, and asks questions that are unanswerable or threatening for the nurse to contemplate.

A nurse's own feelings of love, morality, and marriage are uniquely revealed as she cares for the adolescent seeking and needing sex "information." Therefore, she should be aware that she gives more than facts, no matter how factual, objective, and scientific she tries to make it. She also transmits her own embarrassment or comfort, her fear or antagonism, or her pride in womanhood. Because professional sanction bestows authority, the nurse can be a forceful influence on the adolescent girl. She can be a paragon of warmth and involvement in giving and caring for others or can be one of coldness and noninvolvement. The early experiences of both nurse and patient influence their later interactions. Some of these experiences are presented in this chapter, since they occur to the adolescent girl. By no means all inclusive, they indicate some ways young girls are influenced toward womanhood.

PUBERTY AND THE MENARCHE

These terms are not synonymous. Puberty is the phase of life during which there are many alterations in body structure and function, leading from childhood to maturity. Menarche is the time when menstruation starts. The changes of puberty begin two to three years prior to the menarche. They include development of the breasts and external and internal genital organs and changes in body configuration, height, and psychologic aspects of the individual. Characteristic changes in body shape due to increased fat deposits, in addition to a 2- to 3-inch growth spurt, usually signal that menstruation will begin within two to three years. Maturation of the ovaries is indicated by endocrine changes reflected in the epithelium of the vagina and the uterus. All of these changes are induced by increased pituitary function which activates certain endocrine functions of the adrenal glands and ovaries. Growth of pubic hair (adrenarche) and labia undoubtedly are the result of increased adrenal activity.

Menstruation occurs after the uterus has been prepared by estrogenic stimulation and when the interrelationship between the hypothalamus, pituitary, ovaries, and uterus becomes properly established. Menstruation is periodic bleeding from the uterus. It is associated with certain specific endometrial changes secondary to rhythmic secretions by the ovaries. These produce a cycle of pituitary stimulation, ovulation, corpus luteum formation, maintenance of the endometrium, pituitary inhibition, and corpus luteum and endometrial regression followed by menstruation. *Anovulatory menstruation* is cyclic uterine bleeding in the absence of ovulation.

Menstruation

Menstruation (the menarche) usually begins in the twelfth to fourteenth year, but it may occur as early as the age of 9 years or as late as the age of 17 years. It ceases at the menopause, usually between ages 48 and 52 years. Variability in the so-called normal regular menstrual cycle is the rule. The total length of the cycle varies from 23 to 34 days, with the actual bleeding lasting 3 to 7 days. Ovulation usually precedes menstruation by 14 to 16 days, regardless of the period of amenorrhea prior to this particular period. An average blood loss during a normal period lasting 3 to 7 days has been shown to be 25 ml., with a range of 10 to 55 ml. The average loss of iron is 12 mg.

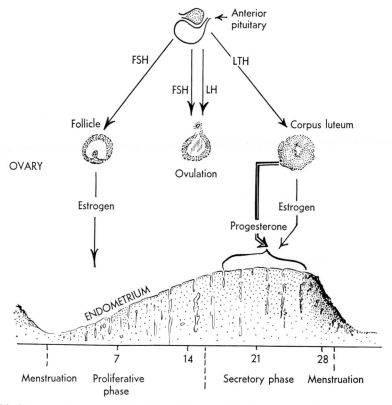

Fig. 2. Pituitary-ovarian-endometrial interrelationships in the menstrual cycle.

Fig. 2 is a schematic diagram showing the pituitary-ovarian-endometrial inter-relationships during a normal menstrual cycle. The diagram shows that the anterior hypophysis (pituitary gland) liberates follicle-stimulating hormone, then luteinizing hormone, and luteotropin (lactogenic hormone). Follicle-stimulating hormone (FSH) acts upon the ovarian follicle and then, in combination with luteinizing hormone (LH), ovulation is induced. Luteotropin (LTH) stimulates the corpus luteum. All these are shown by arrows in Fig. 2. Estrogen originates from the follicle of the ovary and progesterone from the corpus luteum following ovulation. These two hormones act on both the uterine endometrium and on the anterior hypophysis, with estrogen-depressing FSH.

Growth of the endometrium is indicated as the *proliferative phase.* This is a phase during which the endometrium is responding to estrogen. The second phase of the endometrial cycle is termed the *secretory phase,* during which the endometrium responds to both estrogen and progesterone. These hormones prepare the endometrium for the implantation of a fertilized ovum. If pregnancy does not ensue, the corpus luteum regresses, followed by regression of the endometrium and menstruation.

Many experiences of the girl prior to menstruation will influence her attitude toward it. They may be the role of the girl within her family, how she pictures herself within her family group, and the kind of preparation she receives as her physical maturation progresses. Menstruation is considered by some to be a curse, an illness, or a nuisance; others consider it a badge of womanhood or an assurance of normal feminine health. A girl who has been the substitute boy within the family may experience rebellion against a monthly imposition of menstruation and resent any limitation on active competitive sports. The unprepared girl may experience embarrassment, shame, or fear toward menstruation and its monthly recurrence. Inadequate preparation may also perpetuate fear. A student nurse recalls:

> I think I was in seventh grade when I started. All I knew was that you were supposed to be regular and that if you didn't have a period you were pregnant. I didn't understand how a girl became pregnant. When I was irregular for three or four months, I was a very upset individual. I finally found out that periods are often irregular when menstruation begins. I wish I had been told more in the beginning, not just half information.

For the prepared girl, menstruation may mean growing up and becoming a woman, as noted in the statement of another student nurse:

> I can remember when I started and it seems like I was almost proud. I can remember calling Mom to tell her what she'd been expecting for a long time.

Experiences such as these persist in many forms. They many continue in their original feelings, or the negative aspects may become resolved and the positive aspects may mature into a comfortable self-identity. During periods of stress or illness, old attitudes or early experiences sometimes reappear and often are re-experienced within the new context. The nurse experiences her own feelings and remembered incidents. They may be activated or intensified by a patient who reminds her of herself or one who provides the antithesis of her own feelings. It is for this reason that many nurses find gynecologic patients difficult. The nurse may uncomfortably identify with another of her sex if she awakens the nurse's latent feelings or threatens her own present safeness.

The patient or nurse may possess attitudes toward menstruation that are unknown or strange to the other. Such attitudes have a profound influence on hygienic habits, the feminine role, and the ability to communicate with the helping professions or with the patient about gynecologic symptoms.

National groups seem to possess certain unique attitudes toward menstruation and the woman. Individuals within a common society interpret the attitudes of the group in a unique manner of their own. A woman of foreign heritage in the United States may retain remnants of old attitudes, may hold them in combination with others, may *try* to hold conflicting attitudes, or may try to consider them folk beliefs of the past. However, because such beliefs are not open to public scrutiny or evaluation, they sometimes persist from generation to generation in their original form. Varying concentrations of old European influences may be found in family units within urban and rural communities and between certain geographic regions of the United States. They persist in some form in most patients and nurses in the United States. (Professional education may strongly or superficially superimpose still other influences on the nurse.)

Examples of some menstrual attitudes* are presented to indicate their influence in affecting the patient's or nurse's behavior in personal hygiene, her feminine role, and her ability to communicate gynecologic problems. They show some of the sources of prevailing American attitudes. They also indicate new areas of knowledge necessary in order to attain greater understanding between the patient and the helping professions.

Attitudes influencing hygienic habits. Tendencies to possess unique attitudes prevail in all cultures and family groups. For example, the woman in certain nationality groups seeks to induce a heavy and free flow of blood. She believes that the presence of menstrual blood stimulates the flow of more blood. Because of this belief, some women tend to infrequently change sanitary napkins and stained clothing. School and industrial nurses who teach "acceptable" social-hygiene practices in America therefore require an understanding of the practices and beliefs underlying other cultures' hygienic habits. Unless this is understood by those who could help, the individual with European or Asian influences may feel forced to abandon old beliefs for more socially acceptable ideas to which they conform lightly or amidst conflict. For example, an adolescent newly arrived in America

---

*The following discussion on menstrual attitudes is based on the article by Abel, Theodora M., and Joffe, Natalie F.: Cultural backgrounds of female puberty, American Journal of Psychotherapy **4:**90-113, 1950. No follow-up studies since this article was written a generation ago seem to have been made of current influences on the adolescent. The adolescents mentioned in this study are now influencing their own adolescent girls. How?

may feel socially compelled to bathe and change soiled clothing during menstruation. Yet she may still fear the danger to her personal health that she has been taught this practice holds. To resolve the conflicting pressures she may change to a more covert form of sanitary protection and very infrequently change a tampon.

The American girl emphasizes cleanliness during the menstrual period. The American girl, however, may retain a remnant of other nationalities' attitude of the benefits of free menstrual flow when she is cautioned to avoid cold showers and baths.

Many nationalities teach that the menstruating woman is vulnerable during this time. She must be protected from bathing, hair washing, swimming, chills, exercise, and certain kinds of food. These precautions also exist in the United States. A new attitude here warns that teeth should not be filled and that hair is ineffectively permanent waved during the menstrual period. Consider the medical and operative patients in the many clinical areas who coincidently menstruate during their hospitalization. Are patients' behaviors influenced during that time because of certain menstrual beliefs? Does the patient try to avoid bathing, certain foods, or activities? Are these behaviors understood or are they ignored by the helping professions?

Attitudes influencing the feminine role. The beginning of menstruation to some nationalities means the girl's entrance into the society of womanhood. The girl is considered marriageable and physically mature. She is included in women's talk and becomes one of them. That the second- or third-generation American girl seldom feels this strong identity to her sex and proud acceptance by adult women in her new maturity may contribute to the adolescent's feelings of aloneness, competition in society, and an uncertain feminine role.

Some nationality groups believe that the menstruating woman is easily aroused sexually. Therefore, the virgin girl who is menstruating is protected from contact with men and boys. Does this attitude have any later influences on this woman now in the United States? Would she delay or would she seek medical help from male physicians for abnormal bleeding?

The woman's standing in her society during menstruation varies according to nationality. This is often expressed by descriptive language or slang used for menstruation. Folk belief in some nationalities considers the woman dangerous to her family and community during menstruation. Her activity with the family is limited and marital relations are forbidden. Some consider the subject *and* the woman disgusting. Some are extremely secretive and deny its presence. It may be well to consider here that while "sex" is supposedly an open topic in America, menstruation is a subject of embarrassment. What are the effects of these attitudes when they exist in the adolescent girl and the woman in America as she faces gynecologic symptoms and disease? What effect do these attitudes have on routine gynecologic examinations, adolescent examinations, dysmenorrhea, and menopause?

American girls express fear of others' knowledge of their menstruation. This was a common theme in early advertisements for sanitary protection. Its meaning is implied in present-day advertisements. The intensity of this fear of exposure and its effect on adolescent social relationships may be seen in the following student nurse comments:

It can be bad when you're teased by other kids. I can remember a first day when the flow was heavy, and I leaked through. There were a couple of boys walking along behind me and I will never forget nor forgive the teasing that I got on the way home. It makes me worry even now, especially the first couple of days.

I had that same experience but had the fortune of having one of my friends spot it first. We went to the office and called Mom for another change of clothes. It's a terrible feeling of being afraid that you will soil your clothes.

Such experiences can create succeeding attitudes of anxiety or dread with each menstrual cycle. This could be a source of fear or depression that increases the pain experience and induces symptoms of dysmenorrhea. When a nurse knows the availability of extra protective devices, she may advise and help to allay extreme self-consciousness and fears in adolescents and mature women. These are factors to be considered for each patient and for self-knowledge in each nurse as she cares for her patients.

Ability to communicate gynecologic problems. Accurate communication implies accurate perception. It has already been stated that some national groups tend to believe that menstrual blood should freely flow, and they equate the flow with fertility. What effect does the presence of this attitude have in the early recognition of menorrhagia, metrorrhagia, or oligomenorrhea? How accurately does a nurse from such a background evaluate the amount of bleeding present in the woman with metrorrhagia or even in the postoperative gynecologic patient?

How accurate are observations and evaluations of symptoms when the observer considers the subject of menstruation disgusting, embarrassing, or secretive? Will such patients and nurses "play down" the incidence and extent of present symptoms? Will their perception and therefore the content of their communication be distorted and inaccurate?

How free does the American adolescent or the American woman feel in confiding distress to a teacher or employer? If she must be absent from school or work, how difficult is it for her to make necessary explanations or arrangements with her teacher or employer. Reproductive malfunction or gynecologic problems cannot be expressed easily if at all by the adolescent and often only with difficulty to the helping professions. This implies a need of greater communication between the helping professions, educators, and the laity for an awareness of the existing difficulty. It also seems imperative that greater contact be achieved between adolescents and members of the helping professions. The female nurse is an opportune bridge. She can identify with and understand the female adolescent. She can extend to her confidence, trust, and advice, leading to an optimum therapeutic relationship with the medical profession.

These few questions have been raised to indicate another area of patient and nurse individualization during personal interactions. It is also meant to point out the paucity of answers and studies seeking these answers due to prevailing American attitudes on the subject. Yet new nationalities continue to be assimilated within our larger cities. Nurses, especially in these areas, are becoming aware of conflicts in hygienic custom, of the present use of the *crudest* protective devices by some of these women, and of the unhappiness and tragedy that occur when gynecologic problems are ignored or denied. America has been referred to as a melting pot. The implications of this to health attitudes, health practices, and medical treatment have been little explored by the helping professions, especially for those people in transition.

GYNECOLOGIC PROBLEMS OF THE ADOLESCENT

The adolescent girl may require medical treatment for dysmenorrhea, amenorrhea, abnormal bleeding, vaginitis, or congenital anomalies.

In the vast majority of gynecologic diseases the diagnosis may be suggested by the history alone. With the adolescent, a "triple history" is essential for the doctor. By this is meant (1) a history is obtained from the patient with her mother present; (2) a history is obtained from the mother alone and the patient alone; and (3) a history is obtained from a usually overlooked family member—the father. The nurse in the office or in the clinic plays a very important role in maneuvering these separate interview periods with the doctor. The mother is helpful in her description of the patient's problems. By talking to the patient alone, the doctor establishes a necessary patient-doctor relationship. He may also learn what preparation, attitudes, fears, or misinformation the patient may have received from her family and friends. By talking to the father, conflicts and relationships between mother and daughter and father and daughter may become evident.

In addition to the usual physical history the pubertal history is essential in the diagnosis and evaluation of endocrine and menstrual problems. *Precocious puberty* is development of secondary sex characteristics and the occurrence of menstruation prior to the age of 9 years. *Delayed puberty* is inadequate sex development and amenorrhea until the age of 18 years or older. The pubertal history determines the age of development of the nipples (usually 9 and 10 years of age), breasts (usually 10 and 11 years of age), pubic hair and genitalia (usually 11 and 12 years of age), pigmented areolae (usually 12 and 13 years of age), axillary hair, cervical mucus, and the appearance of menarche (usually between 13 and 14 years of age). Another important fact obtained in the history is the growth curve. Usually there is a 2- to 3-inch spurt in height approximately two to three years prior to the menarche. This can be very valuable in evaluating delayed menarche.

Physicians have educated parents to the value of routine adolescent physical examinations, but the vaginal portion of the examination has been neglected. This hesitancy is not due entirely to objections by the parents or the adolescents, but probably by the doctors themselves. Pediatric and adolescent gynecology is insufficiently emphasized in schools and training programs. Recently there is a

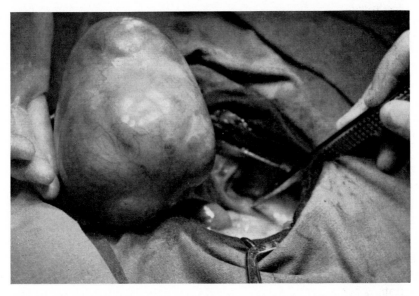

Fig. 3. While unusual in children, this ovarian cyst was found in a 10-year-old girl. The large cyst was twisted and associated with severe abdominal pain prior to operation. This emphasizes the importance of pediatric and adolescent gynecology. (Courtesy Jerome D. Kaufman, Chicago, Ill.)

definite trend toward more training in this area (Fig. 3). If the patient is well prepared prior to examination, and if the physician is gentle and patient, using a few specially designed pediatric instruments, the vaginal examination need be neither difficult nor traumatic for either patient or doctor.

The examination itself begins with a general inspection for evidences of congenital anomalies or abnormal growth. It is followed, as in the adult, by visualization of the vagina, for which there are numerous well-designed instruments. A satisfactory palpation can usually be done vaginally, and if not, a rectal-abdominal examination may be made. This should be explained to the patient prior to the examination. Auxiliary diagnostic procedure includes all those in the adult: wet smear, vaginal cultures, cytosmears, biopsies, and occasional hormone assays.

The presence of the nurse during this examination is important to the adolescent. Unsure of her feelings about sex and denying anything that implies that she is not right, the adolescent needs the understanding of another female—the nurse. Thorough draping throughout the entire examination is more essential for this age group than any other. The position itself will be a strange and embarrassing one for her. If the relationship of trust and confidence exists between the patient, doctor, and nurse, the patient will be more relaxed throughout the examination. A more comprehensive and elucidating examination is possible under such conditions.

Dysmenorrhea

Dysmenorrhea (painful menstruation) is a frequent problem among adolescents.

Primary. Primary or essential dysmenorrhea means the pain had its onset early in menstrual life. The cause of dysmenorrhea is not completely understood and the source of pain is not known. The pain is usually cramplike and more severe during the first two days of menstrual flow. It may be generalized pain in the region of the pelvis, or it may be localized in one pelvic quadrant more than the other. When severe dysmenorrhea exists, pelvic pain, with radiation to the back, thighs, and upper legs, may be experienced. Chills, nausea, and emesis are not uncommon.

Although the etiology of dysmenorrhea is uncertain, factors that influence the processing component of pain (Chapter 2) are very important. It must be emphasized that the family attitude may be extremely helpful or harmful. Dysmenorrhea may occur because of misinformation, misconceptions, or family traditions and fears. When the girl is prepared prior to menarche and is helped during the early months after menarche to understand that menstruation is a normal function, that it may be irregular and uncomfortable, and that activity need not be restricted, the menarche and subsequent menstruation usually produce little psychic or physical disturbance in the individual.

Dysmenorrhea occurring at the onset of menarche and succeeding menstruations may be caused by the presence of congenital anomalies. A rudimentary horn of a double uterus, strictures of the cervix and vagina, partial absence of the vagina, or an imperforate hymen may all be accompanied by severe menstrual pain. Therefore, it is essential that all patients with primary dysmenorrhea be evaluated and examined.

No therapy is used until a complete physical and pelvic examination has ruled out pelvic abnormalities. When this has been assured, treatment may take the form of administered analgesics, sedatives, tranquilizers, or antispasmodics. Less frequently, hormones are prescribed to produce anovulatory cycles, which are theoretically *not* accompanied by pain. The reason for this is unknown. Decreasing detrimental social and psychologic factors through understanding relationships and teaching often provide complete relief.

A contemptuous attitude toward the patient who has dysmenorrhea by one who may or may not have the same problem is not uncommon. The patient may experience her pain as extremely severe. Pain, although arising from a physiologic function common to all women, will necessarily be experienced differently in each individual. This is because of the diversity and uniqueness of individual factors involved in the *processing* component of the pain experience. (The *input* component or the actual arousal of "pain" transmission to the cortex may be similar in most individuals.) The effect of fatigue, fear, and nausea in influencing the pain experience should be remembered. Nursing therefore takes into account all those influences that reduce the pain experience.

Secondary. Secondary or acquired dysmenorrhea has its onset several years after menarche and is often associated with demonstrable organic pelvic lesions. In the adolescent, *primary dysmenorrhea* is more frequent.

Amenorrhea

Amenorrhea is the absence of menstruation. *Primary amenorrhea* is the term used to signify that a girl has not started to menstruate by the age of 17 or 18 years. When a girl has not menstruated by the age of 18 years and has retarded development of secondary sex characteristics, it is considered *delayed menarche.* Such delay may be indicative of some serious abnormality. Therefore, all adolescents who have not menstruated prior to the age of 15 or 16 years should be examined and evaluated. *Secondary amenorrhea* signifies that menstruation has ceased after an individual has previously menstruated normally.

Primary. Variations in the anatomic structure or the physiologic function of the genital organs, the pituitary gland, or other endocrine glands may cause amenorrhea. Congenital anatomic abnormalities such as the absence of the uterus, absence of the ovaries, or obstructions to the outflow of menstrual blood result in amenorrhea. The rare abnormalities of intersex, pseudohermaphroditism, and true hermaphroditism also cause primary amenorrhea. Pituitary tumors as well as ovarian tumors may cause amenorrhea. Endocrine abnormalities, both thyroid and adrenal, must be considered. The adrenogenital syndrome is due to an enzyme deficiency within the adrenal cortex. This results in pseudohermaphroditism if it occurs during the embryonic development of the female. If it has its onset after birth, masculinization and amenorrhea may result. Therefore, a complete examination is essential to rule out congenital anomalies, hormone-producing tumors, or endocrine aberrations of the ovaries, pituitary, thyroid, and adrenal glands.

The diagnosis of these entities is based on general habitus, the history and physical examination, plus special hormone studies and x-ray studies. This means that the adolescent who already fears she is not "normal" is exposed to many examinations and appointments in the office, clinic, or hospital. While this activity tends to reassure an adult and indicates that something is being done to solve a problem, such increased physical attention and its directed focus on illness or abnormal function are very disturbing to the adolescent. The nurturing role of the nurse to such a patient is apparent, whether in the office or hospital outpatient department.

Primary amenorrhea is evaluated and treated according to its etiology. It must be differentiated from delayed menstruation. With a recent growth spurt, it is estimated with relative assurance that menses will begin within two years. If it is "just" delayed menarche in an otherwise normal girl, therapy is based on improving the patient's general health and helping her and her family with the problem.

Problems of amenorrhea in the patient encroach upon the patient's psyche as to the extent of her femaleness and her future role as a wife and mother. Student nurses remember some of these feelings:

> It's terrible. I'm not regular yet and it's just an awful feeling. You have so many wonders. Am I going to be able to have babies? This is the first one and the most important. I think it would be the most wonderful thing in the world to be able to say, "This date and this date I will be starting my period!" I feel for the girl who starts very late and wonders if and when she will menstruate.

I had several friends, one in particular, who didn't start until very late as a senior in high school and another one who had a period every four months. They were very troubled by this. They wondered if they had everything they were supposed to have, or if what's there wasn't working, and all sorts of things. They wondered if they would ever be able to have babies. They also had the feeling that they were just left out and weren't part of the crowd.

I had a friend who didn't start until she was late in her junior year. Everyone said, "Oh, you're so lucky." This just made her feel worse. She worried about it constantly and wouldn't talk about it, but she used to tell me and she'd say, "I wish I wasn't so lucky." She'd been to the doctor who told her that there was nothing wrong with her and not to worry. She was told, "You're very normal," and yet she really wasn't according to the rest of the crowd. It made her very upset.

Trust and confidence in individual members of the helping professions make possible an environment that allows the adolescent to express these fears of being different and that permit the same expressions of fear and questions to be *repeated* without impatience and censure. Until menstruation begins, she will not feel whole and normal, no matter how many reassurances she receives. She really grieves because she is not like others, because she has incomplete physical manifestations of womanhood, and because she fears her future as a functional woman. As in all grief, she requires time, understanding, and the support of her family and the helping professions. An insistence that she verbally state that she, too, knows she is all right and an insistence that she accepts the doctor's reassurance may make it impossible for her to ever again raise questions, doubts, or express her continuing anxiety. The door of communication is closed to her. The nurse in the neighborhood, school, doctor's office, camp, or hospital can provide the understanding and the avenue of communication this adolescent requires. She also may interpret the adolescent's continuing problem and her feelings to her family. Since they may have accepted the doctor's prognosis, they may be completely unaware of or impatient with her continuing worries about herself. In an adolescent such worry and anxiety should be expected.

Secondary. Secondary amenorrhea may occur even in the adolescent. It may be due to such physiologic functions as pregnancy and lactation. Rarely, it may be due to pituitary or various tumors. Other causes may be psychogenic in nature, including pseudocyesis. Secondary amenorrhea is rather commonly seen in adolescents who change schools or who change from home to dormitory living. It is not infrequently present for the first few months in freshmen entering colleges and schools of nursing.

Anxiety about possible pregnancy or fear of unknown causes may continue for many months before this patient finally seeks help. If she is away from home for the first time and knows few people within her new environment, she will be further deterred from seeking help. Sensitivity of the helping professions to adolescents and young adults and *genuine interest* in them permit them to trust. When sincere interest in and sensitivity to others exists, *mutual* trust permits open and honest communication and permits help to be asked for and extended freely and without censure.

Abnormal bleeding

During adolescence abnormal bleeding is seldom associated with tumors. With advancing years, pathologic lesions play a more prominent role in the production of abnormal bleeding. Abnormal bleeding in the adolescent is frequently anovulatory (95%) and is designated *dysfunctional bleeding.* Irregular menses are usual during the early years of menstrual life. If the bleeding occurs too often (less than every 21 days) or if it is profuse, prolonged, or continuous in nature, it must be investigated.

Malignancies, estrogen-producing tumors, benign polyps, and complications of pregnancy may be present in the adolescent patient. Therefore, diagnosis of dysfunctional bleeding is made only after excluding all organic causes. If a satisfactory examination in the office cannot be performed, an examination under anesthesia is necessary, at which time a curettage and biopsy may be performed. A general medical survey, physical examination, cytosmear, blood count, and clotting time are performed to exclude local or systemic disease as causes of the bleeding. If the final diagnosis is dysfunctional bleeding, the treatment consists of iron, vitamins, diet, and hormone therapy. Hormone therapy consists of estrogenic or progestational agents to stop the bleeding. They are then used cyclicly to restore normal menstrual cycles. Hyperthyroid or hypothyroid dysfunction, when present, is treated.

Vaginitis

Probably the most common problem among the adolescent, as in the adult, is vaginal discharge. Although vaginitis occurs frequently, it is disconcerting, uncomfortable, and annoying for all ages of women. The common causes are the nonspecific infections, streptococcus, *Escherichia coli, Candida albicans, Trichomonas vaginalis,* and gonococcus. Foreign-body reactions and foul-smelling vaginal discharge result from objects placed in the vagina, particularly by the younger girl, or a "lost" tampon. Pinworms are also an important cause of vulvovaginitis in younger girls. Diagnostic procedures of examination, wet smears, and cultures are utilized as they are in the adult.

Vaginal discharge is socially unacceptable and frightening to the adolescent. It may disturb her that she is not clean or that she detects an offensive odor despite her efforts of personal hygiene. Pruritus may also be present. As in the adult, pruritus and discharge, singly or in combination, indicate infection to the adolescent patient and perhaps recall vague stories of "social disease" and shame. Because of this, diagnosis and treatment may be delayed because of fear in confiding the condition and its unknown cause to her parents.

Venereal disease

While adolescent sex education seems to be improving through better publications and formal teaching, knowledge of the dangers of venereal diseases and their symptoms remains obscure and repressed by most of the adolescent population.

Yet the greatest increases in the nationwide upswing in the incidence of venereal diseases are within the age group of 13 to 20 years. Venereal diseases constitute the largest communicable disease incidence in the United States.

The child before the age of menarche may contract gonorrhea through an infected adult in the household. Her symptoms are different from an adult's, and the disease does not result in future reproductive complications if it is treated. The adolescent's infection of gonorrhea or syphilis, however, is similar to the adult's. It presents the same symptoms and seriously threatens the future life and happiness of the individual.

Adolescents are influenced through personal example of adult models and the sincere teaching of those felt by the adolescent to be interested in them. Venereal disease holds a moral as well as a physical and social stigma. Nurses in schools, industry, offices, clinics, camps, and hospitals are provided with appropriate and unique opportunities to help the adolescent know about venereal diseases. She is also uniquely able to help the adolescent if she should need medical attention. As a woman and a member of a helping-healing profession, she may not condone, but neither may she condemn. She remains accessible and reachable for any patient who needs her. She may opportunely bridge the gap between the family and patient and the patient and doctor. Understanding relationships created with adolescents before crisis situations sometimes prevent and often minimize the extent of the situation if it does occur. This becomes a nursing role of teacher-counselor-model.

Congenital anomalies

In order to better understand congenital anomalies of the genital tract, a brief summary on the development of the female generative system is pertinent.

Developmental anatomy. The ovary develops alongside the kidney and then decends along the body wall until it reaches its position on the lateral wall of the pelvis. The two embryonic paramesonephric ducts (müllerian) grow down toward the pelvis from their beginning as an *e*vagination of the lining of the coelom near the ovary. The ducts extend from the lateral pelvic wall medially. In the midline they fuse to form a single median duct. The cephalic portions of the paramesonephric ducts that remain separate become the uterine tubes. The median portions fuse to form the uterus and a portion of the vagina. The downward growth of the vaginal canal continues until it meets an *in*vagination from the pelvic floor known as the vestibule. The two cavities, vagina and vestibule, eventually meet (establish communication), although some of the tissue persists at the periphery as the hymen.

Developmental anomalies. Failure of the paramesonephric ducts to fuse anywhere along the midline results in many different conditions of anomaly, all of which are forms of duplication. There may be a double vagina, a double cervix, or a double uterus. There may be two vaginal canals with a single uterus, there may be a single cervix with a double body of the uterus (called a bicornuate

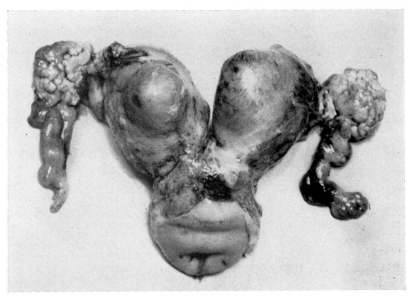

Fig. 4. Single cervix and double body or corpus of the uterus (uterus bicornis unicollis). This uterus was removed from a mature woman, as evidenced by the fact that the specimen reveals the presence of fibroids. The tubes and ovaries are also seen.

uterus, Fig. 4), or there may be a septum dividing the uterine cavity into two portions, with the outside of the uterus appearing as one.

Absence of the vagina and absence of the uterus may result from failure of the downward growth of the paramesonephric ducts. If only the vagina is absent, surgical procedures are possible for construction of an artificial vagina that will connect to the uterus. It allows the patient a normal marital life and a normal reproductive life.

A more common anomaly is the absence of communication between the vagina and the vestibule, resulting in an imperforate hymen. Following menarche, blood is retained in the vagina, and the vagina and uterus soon become distended with blood (hematocolpos and hematometra). The patient has symptoms of a menstrual period, with cramping, but no bleeding. She will not recognize the significance of the symptom since she has never experienced it before. Eventually, a bulging of the vulva and a mass may be felt in the lower abdomen. Treatment consists of incising the septum and allowing the blood to escape. This may be performed in the doctor's office or in the hospital.

Genetic anomalies. Until recent years it was thought that each human cell contained 48 chromosomes. It has now been shown that in the normal cell there are 46 chromosomes: twenty-two pairs of somatic chromosomes and one pair of sex chromosomes. In the female the pair of sex chromosomes is designated as XX and in the male as XY.

Relatively recent advances in diagnostic procedures such as the buccal smear and chromosomal studies are exceedingly valuable in the diagnosis of genetic anomalies. In the diagnosis of Turner's syndrome for ovarian agenesis these two tests have not only demonstrated the diagnosis but also its pathogenesis as a genetic disease. In this syndrome the patients are short, have a webbed neck, a wide carrying angle of the arms, no genital hair, an undeveloped vagina, and no ovarian tissue. Chromosomal studies have shown that Turner's syndrome is a genetic defect, frequently with absence of one X-chromosome. These patients therefore have *45* chromosomes. Their sex chromosome designation is *XO* instead of XX.

Other genetic anomalies exist and may be demonstrated by use of these tests. In Klinefelter's syndrome there is an *extra* complement of chromosomes. Its most common manifestation is *47* chromosomes, with sex chromosomes of XXY. Since these original descriptions, many varied patterns of chromosome counts and combinations have been described and they constitute varying genetic anomaly syndromes.

HOSPITALIZATION OF THE ADOLESCENT

Hospitalization is especially difficult for the adolescent. The necessity of medical or surgical treatment forces the adolescent to focus on physical feelings, illness, and separation from her peers and family. All these seem to imply that she is different and therefore isolated from the peer group, which usually gives the adolescent some measure of security. A congenital anomaly involving reproductive organs isolates the adolescent from the "club" of young womanhood. If she does not menstruate, she may be isolated from girl talk and confidences. Her peers may exclude her or the patient herself may retreat from their conversation in embarrassment and shame.

When the hospitalization itself is necessary, she is faced with a dilemma. *How* can she explain her absence from school and friends? Even if "sex" is a common conversation, personal disease, gynecology, or abnormality is *not* adolescent conversation. Even if the patient has said nothing to her friends, she may still be uneasy and worried. "If only they won't find out." "What if they do and they come to the hospital." These kinds of thoughts become nightmares for the patient. What are the effects of such dread on the postoperative convalescent course? What are the effects of visits of the peers or the effects of adolescent or adult roommates in the hospital with an adolescent gynecologic patient? How does the nurse herself feel about a gynecologic anomaly and the increased emphasis placed on it by the operative therapy itself? How does she affect the patient? How does the family feel? These are a few of the inquiring probes that should trouble every nurse as she tries to help each particular patient.

There is still a certain shame or guilt associated with congenital anomalies. Often there is scrutiny on both sides of the family for "the blame." In addition, the conditions surrounding the pregnancy and the desirability of the pregnancy are often reconsidered and pondered when an anomaly of any kind is discovered. If the anomaly was discovered earlier in the patient's life and operative treatment delayed until adolescence, the feelings of guilt or shame in the family may again become aroused and intensified by the operative event. For this reason, both the patient and her family require help during the operative period. Because of their detachment from the threatening biologic aspects of the hospitalization, hospital social workers often are important adjuncts to the helping professions concerned with this patient and her family.

Congenital anomalies of the genital tract also concern the nurses caring for the patient. Although seldom acknowledged by the nurse, congenital anomaly often bears the stigma of the "sins of the fathers." In addition, it involves the reproductive organs and therefore the context of femininity. Therefore, the nurse may practice a certain safe physical or psychologic distance from the patient who makes her feel uncomfortable. She may experience pity and a feeling of "I'm glad I'm not like her." This is really an expression of superiority to a patient who is "crippled" or deficient, and it only increases the distance between effective nurse-patient understanding. "Superiority" feelings are fostered when the nurse's vulnerable feelings of fear cannot be safely expressed and when therapeutic interpersonal relationships between the nurse and patient are avoided because of feared "involvement."

Placement of the adolescent in the clinical unit should be of great importance to all concerned with the welfare of the patient. To admit the adolescent to the pediatric area implies to the adolescent that the hospital and those in it consider and respect her no more than a "kid." The incongruence of the action is especially apparent when the adolescent, laden with her uneasy feelings about sex, is admitted to pediatrics for gynecologic problems.

To admit the adolescent to the general clinical units with adult patients presents further problems. Illness and death are especially frightening to the adolescent, for it focuses her attention on her body and its functions and emphasizes her inability to be in control of herself and mounting threats to her health. While a nurse often has little influence on the hospital admitting procedure unless she is in an administrative position, the nurse in the clinical unit can be cognizant and alert to this predicament of the adolescent. She *can* rescue the adolescent from a detrimental room placement with a frightening senile patient, an irrational patient, an acutely ill patient, a terminally ill patient, or one with mutilating surgery such as extremity amputations, colostomy, mastectomy, or radical neck resection.

With increasing interest in adolescent medicine, perhaps the day is not distant when all hospitals will consider an adolescent clinical unit and outpatient department necessary facilities. Such facilities would enhance optimum development of the adolescent toward her own positive health and her own feelings of respect, preservation of modesty, and cooperation in her own hospital recovery. The adolescent seeks self-identity and acceptance by others. This means that *personal attention must be paid to her,* not only to her symptoms and treatment. The adolescent extended personal recognition and trust will least seek to assert her independence in unrealistic situations just to assert herself and prove herself. She *can be helped* to assume independence of action and decision within many aspects of her hospitalization. By example, she can learn to trust an *inter*dependent relationship and suffer no loss of pride, self-worth, or independence. The touch stone is *interest* in and *fidelity* to a changeable individual—the adolescent.

RECOMMENDED READINGS FOR STUDENTS' USE WITH PATIENTS

Guides for strengthening family life in the home, in the community, in the schools, in health and social agencies, New York, no date. American Social Health Association. (An annotated bibliography of many books and pamphlets available singly and in quantity. They are categorized as follows: for parents and the growing child; especially for teenagers; for the young adult; and for teachers, social workers, health workers and community leaders. Some pamphlets are available in foreign languages.)

Lerrigo, Marion O., and Southard, Helen: Approaching adulthood, Chicago and Washington, D. C., 1961, American Medical Association and The National Education Association. (Ages 16 to 20 years.)

Lerrigo, Marion O., and Southard, Helen: Finding yourself, Chicago and Washington, D. C., 1961, American Medical Association and The National Education Association. (Junior high school level.)

Lerrigo, Marion O., and Southard, Helen: A story about you, Chicago and Washington, D. C., 1962, American Medical Association and The National Education Association. (Grades 4 to 6.)

Lerrigo, Marion O., and Southard, Helen: Facts aren't enough, Chicago and Washington, D. C., 1962, American Medical Association and The National Education Association. (For adult education in preparation for teaching youths.)

Publications to help parents in fostering the healthy development of children from birth through adolescence, New York, 1963, Child Study Association of America, Inc. (An annotated bibliography of pamphlets and books.)

Williams, Mary McGee, and Kane, Irene: On becoming a woman, New York, 1960, Dell Publishing Co., Inc.

Teaching aids

Educational portfolio on menstrual hygiene, Milltown, N. J., no date, Personal Products Corporation, Department A. (Booklets and chart with teaching guide.)

From fiction to fact, a teacher's guide on menstruation and menstrual health, New York, no date, Tampax, Inc., Educational Department. (Guide, booklets, and reprints available.)

Helpful teaching aids, Neenah, Wisconsin, 1960, Kimberly-Clark Corporation, Educational Department. (Booklets and film available for teaching to different age groups. Some available in Spanish, French, Chinese, and braille.)

RECOMMENDED READINGS FOR INSTRUCTORS

Brewer, John I.: Textbook of Gynecology, Baltimore, 1961, The Williams & Wilkins Co., Part I, Section I.

Erikson, Erik, editor: Youth: change and challenge, New York, 1963, Basic Books, Inc., Publishers. Also in Youth: change and challenge, Daedalus, Winter, 1962. (Contributors are Bruno Bettelheim, Reuel Denney, S. N. Eisenstadt, Erik Erikson, Kenneth Keniston, Robert Lifton, Kaspar Naegele, Talcott Parsons, George Sherman, and Laurence Wylie.)

Gallagher, J. Roswell: Medical care of the adolescent, New York, 1960, Appleton-Century-Crofts, Inc., pp. 190-231.

Huffman, J. W., editor: Pediatric gynecology, Clinical Obstetrics and Gynecology 3:133-257, 1960.

Miller, O. J.: The sex chromosome anomalies, American Journal of Obstetrics and Gynecology 90:1078-1139, 1964.

Film

The physiology of normal menstruation, Bloomfield, N. J., Audio-Visual Department, Schering Corporation. (Full color, sound and silent film, 22 and 30 minute running time.)

TYPICAL READINGS ACCESSIBLE TO PATIENTS

Bauer, W. W., and Bauer, Florence Marvyne: Those difficult years of change, Today's Health **43**(3):46-49, 89, 1965.

Beck, Jean: The big question for teens: morality, Today's Health **43**(5):23-33, 1965.

Lewis, Donald W.: An emerging specialty: adolescent medicine, Today's Health **43**(2):39-41, 1965.

My problem and how I solved it: How I learned to answer the questions my daughter couldn't ask me, Good Housekeeping **157**(2):10, 12, 16, 18, 1962.

My problem and how I solved it: Our daughter grew up too fast, Good Housekeeping **159**(1): 10, 15, 19-20, 22, 22b, 1964.

Naismith, Grace: Why men should know more about menstruation, Today's Health **41**(9): 22-23, 57-60, 1963.

"Pap" tests for teens, Good Housekeeping **160**(4):24, 1965.

What a girl should know about her first gynecological checkup, Good Housekeeping **160** (3):183, 1965.

Chapter 6

The mature patient

Modern woman has been variously analyzed as an addicted joiner of organizations, a part-time wife and mother, a searcher for happiness and fulfillment, a discontent, an associate and equal, an emancipated hausfrau, and a polyglot of fragmented ambitions, activities, and responsibilities that yield transitory satisfactions. She often interrupts her education for marriage and shares many of her years of marriage with a job which she seeks for "money, identity, achievement, status, personal pride, inner joy, and . . . a lasting peace rather than a cease-fire within marriage."* She bears large families, sometimes experiences pride in breast feeding, involves her family in community participation, and jealously guards their present and future security in that community.

She is both present and future oriented, sometimes preferring the known present to the nebulous dangers of the future and sometimes rushing the future to escape the doldrums of the present. She may rush preadolescent dating and adolescent pseudoadult activity but hold back the future that forewarns her physical changes, her husband's aging, and changing family roles. She values newness, youth, beauty, vitality, abundance, and fecundity. In many instances she is as uncomfortable and inexperienced in the presence of illness in others and herself as is the adolescent. The possibility of death is considered, if thought of at all, as remote; the eventuality of death belongs to the distant generation of the grandparent and, later, the parent. She assumes that they look forward to and have little fear of death. Illness is abnormal; hospital care is for the ill. She often fears involvement, physical as well as emotional.

The presence or absence of these orientations or values is an individual variation. Some are present in many American middle class women; some are absent in

---

*Rostow, Edna G.: Conflict and accommodation. In The woman in America, Daedalus, Spring, 1964, p. 748.

many women. Their presence or absence in the woman seeking help from the healing professions will influence the time and way in which the help is sought. Their presence or absence will influence the extent and manner in which help is extended to her by others. Communication is profoundly affected in the sender and receiver.

Any basic consideration of the mature woman involves who she thinks she is. Her mold of womanhood is set by her mother and the other women (aunts, grandmothers, etc.) who raised her. It is set by her relationship with her father and her interpretation of other men as kind, strong, wise, fierce, etc. It is set by the model of her parents' relationship. Whether a woman is proud and comfortable with her sex or whether she is not becomes a very important factor when the woman becomes a gynecologic patient.

Increasing concern is being focused on the similarity of the sexes in career roles and on the growing similarity of the father and mother in their home work roles. In many occupations now held by women aggressive action and drive are essentials. In other jobs women's work has been described as "repetitive drudgery, related to *things* rather than to people."* Yet "through the ages, human beings have remained human because there were women who provided continuity in their lives . . . to be there when they woke up, to ease pain, to sympathize with failure and rejoice at success, to listen to tales of broken hearts, to soothe and support and sustain and stimulate husbands and sons as they faced the vicissitudes of a hard outside world. Who in the population will now be *free* to care . . .?"*

Women, more than men, are the creators and nourishers of mankind. They give, and they seem to find their wellspring of renewed strength in contemplative inward turning. Surrounded by multitudes of demands on their time and energies, many of them insignificant, modern women find it increasingly difficult to become renewed with inner strength. Mature woman is measured by her sincere concern in others first, particularly her family, and herself later. She desires to give completely. This she is unable to do until she is able to achieve restoration through spiritual, esthetic, or creative sources.† Mature woman is interdependent: as with every individual, she must receive in order to give.

The meaning of life, her place in it, and who she thinks she is are crucial meditations for the young mature woman who grows through her relationships of marriage, the early family, and the community. These are necessary contemplations for the nurse, whose function also is to nurture. They are necessary contemplations to reevaluate and to mature as the woman's roles and life changes. They enable her to develop and to grow from early family relationships to ones that involve the inclusion of strangers into the intimate family unit, a diminution of her family's responsibilities, and a growing interest in the future generations.

---

*Meade, Margaret: An appraisal of the Report by the President's Commission on the Status of Women, Redbook Magazine, November, 1963.

†Lindbergh, Anne Morrow: Gift from the sea, New York, 1955, Pantheon Books, Inc.

Premenopausal, menopausal, and climacteric depression, doubts, and self-depreciation are infrequent when women recognize and plan for their changing environment and when they know and respect themselves within it. Sometimes they require help to understand their husband and other family members affected by the changes as the family enlarges, grows, and leaves for school, marriage, and the founding of a new family unit. The helping-healing professions are often sought for guidance. The gynecologic patient seems greater perturbed by family relationships and roles than other patients seeking medical advice. Her symptoms and the way she relates them are often combined and interrelated to the degree of her social and emotional well-being.

Gynecologic patients are often *self*-interested and *self*-concerned. They are ill and seek help from the healing professions. Yet self-concern in a woman in the absence of her expected concern for others is little tolerated by other women. The nurse gives freely to the *self*-concerned male patient and to the *self*-centered child or adolescent. She often feels constraint and antagonism toward evidences of a *self*-concerned woman. Even in illness, apparently, a woman is expected to give, not overtly request and receive. Demanding, whining, self-pitying, and *self*ish describe nurses' stated feelings toward the woman patient. When the woman is threatened by disorders of the reproductive organs or of their function, she seems to be less accepted, understood, and nurtured.

Only a small proportion (5 to 10%) of gynecologic patients require operative treatment. "Medical gynecology" or "office gynecology" has assumed vast importance due to the expanding developments in bacteriology, psychiatry, reproductive physiology, and endocrinology. The gynecologist is a combination internist, psychiatrist, physiologist, and specialized surgeon. Because of the intimate nature of gynecologic problems, the quality of the doctor-patient-nurse relationship will influence the confidence and trust of the patient, the accuracy of the history given, the diagnosis, and the effect of the therapy.

GYNECOLOGIC PROBLEMS OF THE MATURE WOMAN

Although the patient often presents herself for a "routine checkup," symptoms of leukorrhea with itching, abnormal uterine bleeding, pelvic pain, and dysmenorrhea are frequent complaints of gynecologic patients. A variety of other symptoms may bring the patient to the doctor. These include developmental anomalies, amenorrhea, infertility, infections, and incontinence.

Gynecologic physical examination

An accurate history is essential. The majority of gynecologic diseases can be diagnosed or suggested by the history alone. It has been said that "history taking is an art," particularly when the gynecologic patient may be reluctant to tell the intimate details of her problem. In addition to the patient's main symptoms and the history of present illness, the menstrual and obstetric history, previous illnesses, operations, and any pertinent family history are important in making an accurate diagnosis. Many systemic diseases may manifest themselves as gynecologic symptoms. Many gynecologic diseases, particularly malignancies and endocrinopathies, may have systemic effects.

The general physical examination includes blood pressure, pulse, and temperature. Examination of the breasts is very important. The abdomen is also examined. Pelvic examination begins with gross inspection of the external genitalia. This may reveal anatomic abnormalities, irritations, relaxation lesions, tumors, or bleeding. The speculum examination, with visualization of the cervix, is performed on all patients. For those very young or those with an intact hymen, special instruments are used. This is followed by a cytosmear for malignancy and may also include studies of cervical mucus and vaginal epithelium for hormonal abnormalities. These are best obtained under direct vision by the use of a speculum. The cytosmear (Papanicolaou smear) is performed on every patient. This is a simple procedure, performed merely by taking a cervical scraping or specimen from the vagina, putting it on a slide, and fixing it in alcohol. It is later stained and examined microscopically. An abnormal smear, indicating possible malignant cells, means that further diagnostic procedures must be done. A patient is never treated on the basis of the results of the cytosmear alone. The examination is completed with a bimanual examination of the pelvis to determine the size, shape, consistency, mobility, and position of the uterus, tubes, and ovaries.

Many lesions are missed if palpation alone is relied on; cervicitis and polyps may not be felt and carcinoma may be overlooked. It is also impossible to diagnose early carcinoma of the cervix by visual means only. A *complete gynecologic examination* includes direct visualization of the cervix, a bimanual examination, and a cytosmear.

Pain and discomfort will be experienced by the patient in the presence of anxiety, embarrassment, and fear. However, even in the presence of tender pelvic lesions, the examination may cause little discomfort when it has been preceded by the explanations and considerate preparations of the nurse and doctor and performed with gentleness and reassurances. Some doctors prefer a nurse to be present in the examining room. The nurse can help the patient during the examination to reduce her apprehensions and to relax during the examination. Discomfort will be minimized. The nurse's function is therefore beneficial to both patient and doctor. Her "job" as only a hander of instruments can be eliminated for her more important role by the convenient placement of instruments and equipment for the doctor's use. (More extensive discussion of the importance of the nurse-doctor-patient interaction prior to and during the examination may be found in Chapter 3.)

Abnormal uterine bleeding

Abnormal uterine bleeding is a common symptom in the mature years of a woman's life. During adolescence it is seldom associated with tumors. With advancing years, pathologic lesions play a more prominent role in production of bleeding. Abnormal uterine bleeding means excessive, prolonged, too frequent menstrual cycles, intermenstrual spotting, or continuous bleeding. Any bleeding that is different from that which a particular patient is accustomed should be considered abnormal.

To properly treat abnormal bleeding the doctor must first make an accurate diagnosis. It is essential to ascertain the source of the bleeding. Often patients note blood in the toilet or on the tissue and erroneously assume it is of uterine or vaginal origin. The doctor must be sure that the blood has not arisen from the vulva, the bladder, the rectum, or the vagina. If blood is found in these regions, he does not conclude that the uterus is free of disease. It is possible, for example, that there may be bleeding from either a urethral caruncle or a cervical polyp and bleeding from the uterus at the same time. The latter might be indicative of a serious lesion such as a uterine malignancy. A complete gynecologic examination is essential.

No patient with abnormal uterine bleeding should be treated until every practical method of determining its cause has been utilized. Abnormal uterine bleeding may be due to local or systemic factors. Bleeding in women of the childbearing age is considered a complication of pregnancy until proved otherwise. This may be the complication of threatened abortion, ectopic pregnancy, hydatid mole, or even choriocarcinoma. Other causes of bleeding from the uterus include benign and malignant tumors of the cervix and body of the uterus; fibroids, adenomyosis, endometrial and cervical carcinoma, or sarcoma; inflammatory lesions of the cervix and endometrium; pelvic inflammatory disease; polyps of the cervix or endometrium (Fig. 5); certain ovarian tumors; or dysfunctional bleeding. (See Fig. 1.) It may be due to other causes such as exogenous hormones, bleeding following trauma, or slight spotting at the time of ovulation. Uterine bleeding may be due to systemic factors. Approximately 10% of patients with systemic hemorrhagic diseases have abnormal uterine bleeding. Hemorrhagic disease is suspected when uterine bleeding coexists with other bleeding tendencies such as petechiae, ecchymoses, bruising easily, or frequent epistaxis. The leukemic patient is included in this group. To an adolescent or woman the presence or cessation of uterine bleeding becomes a measure of her condition. Though she may have many other visible sites of bleeding, uterine bleeding portends to her the length of her future.

If, after complete investigation, no cause can be found for abnormal bleeding, then and only then can it be classified as "dysfunctional uterine bleeding."

Dysfunctional uterine bleeding. Dysfunctional uterine bleeding is almost as difficult to define as it is to cure. It is considered to be abnormal bleeding persisting for a period of time for which a cause cannot be found. Usually the bleeding is associated with failure of ovulation, with a prolonged estrogen phase. Treatment depends on the severity of the symptoms, the age of the patient, the number of children, and her desire for future pregnancies. Curettage is frequently both diagnostic and curative. It is frequently performed in patients with dysfunctional bleeding, particularly those who have associated anemia. Following curettage, it is safe

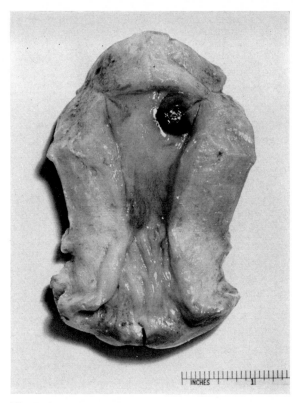

Fig. 5. An endometrial polyp.

to use hormone therapy. In women who are past the age of 35 years, have their family, and have not improved with medical treatment, hysterectomy may be the treatment of choice.

This patient depends on a strong relationship with the doctor. With increased flow or frequent periods of bleeding, the patient requires trust in the ability of her doctor and patience to await the results and evaluation of the diagnostic procedures. She may be required to enter the hospital for a curettement, a minor procedure to the hospital personnel but a major procedure and family disruption to the patient. She has no assurance that the procedure in itself will be therapeutic or that further operative procedures will not be indicated. She faces the possibility of a diagnosis of cancer. After discharge from the hospital, if the curettement did not change the bleeding pattern, the patient's apprehensions and fears of malignancy return. Fear of soiling and the offensive odor of the blood are difficult factors for the woman to cope with as she tries to work or entertain socially.

Until the final therapy is evaluated and prescribed, the waiting and indecision require that *someone* help her. If *someone* does not, the patient is often unable to function as fully as she wants to for her family; she is often physically tired and concerned for herself, her family, and a nebulous future. She may be unable to communicate her concern to any of her family or friends. It is often even easier to express pain than the presence of profuse uterine bleeding. The nurse in industry, public health, or the doctor's office can give her understanding and support, thereby helping her to continue to give to her family despite self-worry. The neighbor or friend who is a nurse could also "give" to her.

Complications of early pregnancy. In any woman of childbearing age abnormal uterine bleeding first suggests a complication of early pregnancy; abortion or ectopic gestation is the most common. Abortion is the expulsion of the contents of the pregnant uterus prior to 20 weeks' gestation. *Miscarriage* is the lay term used for this condition. Abortion suggests something illegal to the average person. In medical usage there is no such implication. This implies that the word "abortion" should be used with caution in obtaining a preliminary history from the patient or in referring to her diagnosis *unless* the medical use of the word is explained to her and its criminal connotation deleted. Even so, friends and family may react to the use of this word within their presence and the patient's. Abortions may be spontaneous or induced. Spontaneous abortion occurs in 10 to 20% of all pregnancies and may be due to several causes. The most common is abnormality of the ovum itself, so that an actual fetus is not found. Other causes, none of which are proved, may be due to diet, hormonal imbalance, or anatomic abnormalities or related to systemic diseases. Acute infectious diseases may cause abortion.

A single spontaneous abortion does not indicate any gynecologic concern, but subsequent abortions give rise to increasing concern. Three consecutive spontaneous abortions are termed *habitual abortion*. Numerous modes of treatment have been proposed. Prenatal care that accents nutrition, rest, and general medical well-being results in a high rate of term pregnancies. Congenital anomalies such as a double uterus or rudimentary horn have been associated with repeated abortions; multiple uterine fibroids are also associated with repeated abortions. Although unusual, a syndrome known as the "incompetent cervical os" has received a great deal of publicity in recent years. In this syndrome the cervix, either due to a congenital weakness or to trauma of previous deliveries or surgical procedures, dilates painlessly during the second trimester of pregnancy and spontaneous abortion or immature delivery occurs. A surgical procedure known as the Shirodkar operation or cervical circlage has been developed in which a string of nylon, fascia, or suture is placed around the cervix submucously and tied tightly to prevent the cervix from dilating prematurely. When properly indicated, this operation results in a high percentage of term or viable pregnancies.

It is important that all nursing and auxiliary personnel understand what this operation is and that they *all* know whenever a newly admitted patient has had this operation. The patient herself should know the importance of early recognition and reporting of labor. Public health and industrial nurses should also be cognizant of this operation and what it means. Danger of a ruptured uterus is imminent when any type of obstructed labor exists. As soon as *early* labor *begins,* the attending doctor should be notified at once. He will cut the suture and labor will be allowed to proceed, or delivery will be accomplished promptly by cesarean section.

Any woman in the first 20 weeks of pregnancy who bleeds vaginally is considered to have a *threatened abortion*. Usually this subsides and the pregnancy continues to term. On the other hand, it may proceed to an *inevitable abortion,* in which there is cramping pain of uterine contractions, cervical effacement, and dilatation. Usually the embryo is already dead or some abnormality of the ovum exists that is incompatible with continuing the pregnancy. When a portion of the uterine contents has been expelled, it is known as an *incomplete abortion;* when the entire contents have been expelled, it is considered a *complete abortion*. In all cases it is important to determine what has been passed, either the whole ovum, with its surrounding placenta and decidua, or only blood clots. All blood clots should therefore be retained for gross inspection. Hospitalized patients should use only a bedpan or commode, so that all tissue passed may be inspected. The bleeding patient at home is best advised to use a bedpan or commode instead of the toilet during this time.

Threatened abortions are treated by rest and precautionary measures such as sedatives. The value of hormones, particularly progesterone, is regarded as doubtful.

Incomplete abortion, which is characterized by dilation of the cervix and passage of a portion of the products of conception, is usually managed by surgical evacuation—curettage. If there is no bleeding and if the entire products of conception have been expelled, observation may be all that is necessary.

In *septic abortion* the contents of the uterus have become infected. Today this is one of the most important causes of maternal death. Antibiotics early and in adequate doses are essential. If the abortion is still incomplete, the evacuation of the remaining contents is a matter of judgment. The risk of operative interference and disseminating infection against the removal of the mass of infected placental debris that is the source of systemic infection must be weighed. In these patients severe complications of bacteremic or endotoxin shock may occur. Therefore, great vigilance is necessary, with particular attention to the vital signs of blood pressure and pulse as well as to the amount of bleeding. Any increase in bleeding or a rise of temperature (which on occasion may go as high as 105° F.) or blood pressure which indicates impending shock should, of course, be reported immediately. The mortality in these patients is extremely high. They must be treated with large doses of antibiotics and steroids, fluid replacement, and evacuation of the infected contents of the uterus. A patient who enters the hospital with a simple incomplete abortion for "just a D & C" may become a tragic maternal death in a few minutes' time unless the vigilance and judgment of the nursing and medical house staff are maintained at all times.

For the hospital personnel, a patient's mourning for a lost fetus may seem out of proportion to the situation, especially if it is lost early in the pregnancy. However, it is not unusual for the mother to mourn for the potential future of the individual and for her plans and future.

The loss of life itself is seldom considered lightly by the family. This is especially true if the conception occurred after the death of another child or before the injury or death of the father. Even in the absence of such sorrows, an interruption of a pregnancy more than a few months old ruins plans, hopes, and anticipations of a new family member. The symptoms of grief in the patient are usual. She needs those who are understanding and sensitive to her grief. The patient may also experience feelings of failure. This may be especially prevalent in the woman who has had a recurrence of abortions. She may feel herself an unsatisfactory woman and bearer of a child for her family or her husband. If she had hopes of a pregnancy cementing a shaky marital relationship, the abortive action may have greater significance to her than the loss of the fetus. It may mean the loss of her marriage.

Because these patients seldom look ill and are soon up and ready to go home, custodial care is common. Nursing involves concern with the patient's physiologic adjustments after an abortive pregnancy and with her emotional redirection after the months of anticipating a successful birth. Emotional upheaval is also experienced by the woman who has spontaneously aborted a fetus that she did not want. Her feelings about the pregnancy, in combination with the loss of the fetus, may arouse guilt, remorse, or relief.

Therapeutic abortion is the deliberate termination of a pregnancy in order to save or safeguard the life or health of the mother. The decision is reached only after consultation between responsible physicians. The procedure is carried out in the operating room with full aseptic precautions. Severe renal disease, late and complicated heart disease, severe psychiatric problems with suicidal tendencies, and rubella infection in the first trimester of pregnancy are some of the more common indications for therapeutic abortion.

Abortion attempted by drugs or instrumentation without legal indications as defined by various state laws, in or not in a hospital, is considered a *criminal* abortion. Associated with it is the risk of infection, hemorrhage, and death. When the individuals of the helping professions are accessible and open in their relationships with others, including the adolescent and young adult, in the neighborhood, church, club, camp, school, or industry, they may become potential sources of guidance and help to troubled and often guilt-ridden adolescents. A knowledge of community resources for financial and maternity care of the unwed pregnant adolescent and woman should be in the possession of *all* nurses, not only public health nurses and social workers. Early help and guidance when initially sought and extended with understanding and sensitivity toward that individual may prevent her frenzied decision for a criminal abortion and a possible loss of two lives. She can be extended help in the midst of her depreciated feelings of social and moral isolation.

Ectopic pregnancy (extrauterine). Ectopic pregnancy is any pregnancy that is implanted elsewhere than in the endometrial cavity. These may be in the uterine tube (called tubal pregnancy), or rarely they may occur in the ovary or in the abdominal cavity itself.

Tubal pregnancy is the most common site. In tubal pregnancy the fertilized

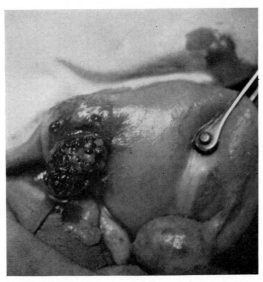

Fig. 6. A ruptured tubal pregnancy. The products of conception may be seen protruding through the wall of the left tube. The other tube and ovary in the foreground are normal.

ovum implants itself in the mucous membrane of the uterine tube. Subsequent changes in the tissue attempt to duplicate the tissue changes in the uterus after a normal implantation. The tube enlarges to accommodate the developing pregnancy, but eventually, usually in the second month of pregnancy, internal hemorrhage occurs, since the tube cannot continue to sustain this unusual function. Tubal rupture occurs with internal abdominal hemorrhage (Fig. 6). Occasionally tubal abortion occurs in which the gestational contents are extruded through the fimbriated end into the peritoneal cavity.

Clinically, a patient may have missed one or two periods. (The endometrium has responded as though the ovum had implanted normally.) As the tubal placenta is disrupted and hormonal changes occur, the patient has uterine bleeding, with the shedding of the decidual cast.

The degree of abdominal pain a patient has depends on the amount of internal hemorrhage. It may be sudden and severe. The patient is acutely ill, may collapse, and appears in shock. The abdomen is rigid and tender. In other patients the history may be the same, but the pain may be intermittent, with less tenderness and rigidity. While the original pain is located in the pelvis, supraclavicular and subdiaphragmatic pain may also be experienced. On examination, movement of the cervix produces pain and tenderness and a mass may be palpated in the adnexa.

An ectopic pregnancy must be differentiated from the medical problems of threatened abortion, incomplete intrauterine abortion, acute salpingitis, persistent corpus luteum cyst, or appendicitis. Biologic pregnancy tests may not be a reliable diagnostic tool during this early stage of a pregnancy. Various other procedures are used to diagnose an ectopic pregnancy. *Colpotomy,* an incision into the cul-de-sac, actually visualizes the tubal gestation for diagnosis. *Culdocentesis* is the insertion of a needle into the cul-de-sac. The withdrawal of blood indicates probable ectopic pregnancy. *Culdoscopy* is the insertion of an instrument to visualize the peritoneal contents so that blood or an actual tubal pregnancy may be seen. When the patient's history and the physical findings suggest ectopic pregnancy, the treatment involves an immediate abdominal laparotomy and removal of the affected tube. Sometimes when the tubal pregnancy has been diagnosed in its unruptured form, the tube simply is surgically opened, the pregnancy removed, and the tube repaired in an effort to retain its reproductive function. Unfortunately, if the original cause of the tubal pregnancy was tubal disease, this patient would be subject to repeated tubal pregnancies.

While uterine abortion and interrupted ectopic pregnancy terminate the pregnancy, the reactions of the patients are often different. The woman with an ectopic pregnancy may be suddenly a very acutely ill patient. She may have suspected pregnancy, or she may as yet have been unaware of its presence. The cause of her symptoms and their significance may be unknown to her.

Immediate hospitalization creates emergency tensions within the home that are absorbed by even the very youngest member of the family. The woman may be torn between the imperative haste necessary for her welfare and the unfulfilled family care or the hardships that her unprepared absence imposes on her family. Her husband may be out of town, relatives must be notified, and the children may be consigned to the care of neighbors or friends, some of whom may not be her choices. While it is impossible for the nurse to resolve any of these stresses for the patient, her ability to protect and to "neutralize" the patient's hospital environment will help the patient. She is aware of the presence of bleeding or shock and the patient's responses to the stresses of bleeding and pain by evaluations of vital signs and other observations. She recognizes the possible presence of many of the patient's unspoken anxieties about home, her family, herself, herself and her family, the hospitalization, operation, and many others. Haste, loud noises, or excited voices accentuate all existing stress factors. The measure of nursing to this patient can be reckoned by the level of confidence and trust a patient can extend to a nurse within their short relationship before the operation. Because the patient has had little time to prepare herself for an operation, she may require postoperative time to realize what has happened to her, why, and what will happen now. Because she was forced to leave her family without preparation for them (she may feel as though she abandoned them), she may express early anxieties about their welfare. She may express this immediately after anesthesia arousal to her husband or to the nurse, even though after the period of extreme stress concern for self-preservation is usual.

Help extended to the husband at this time so that he may reevaluate the family situation and make modifications may not be readily identified as nursing. It may be recalled that any anxiety- or fear-producing situation allowed to proceed unabated may be considered detrimental to the patient's healing process. It may also be recalled that nursing is nurture to the patient or to those who affect her. It then may be accepted that those acts that lighten the family situation and those acts that enhance the healing environment (physical or emotional, internal or external) become nursing to the patient.

Concern for his wife may narrow the husband's perception of the home condition and his ability to give his usual measure of attention and love to the children. The nurse may also help him to understand this dimension. At this time he may find it easier to give his attention and love to the children through their mutual sharing of home activities: together they may perform some of the mother's tasks; together they may purchase flowers for the hospital; and he may encourage them to talk with the mother by telephone or to write notes with enclosed crayon drawings. Because his primary focus is on the wife and mother, he needs help to encompass the children and their changing welfare. Often a social worker is necessary to evaluate the boarding arrangements for the children and to help the husband to determine alternative plans. As the patient's strength is restored and discharge is contemplated, she may be helped to understand the possible responses of children of various ages in periods of emergency illness—the very young child, the 10-year-old boy, or the adolescent. She may then reenter her home with her usual focus of giving to those who need her, even though her physical giving may be curtailed.

Uterine myomas. Uterine myomas are the most frequent uterine tumors. Descriptive terms that portray the tissue components of this new growth are also used, such as fibroid, fibromyoma, or leiomyoma.

Myomas are usually multiple and vary in size from those that are microscopic to those that fill the entire abdominal cavity. They are benign, spherical in shape, and can be easily shelled out, as if actually in a capsule. These tumors first appear during the childbearing period of life and their growth is most often very slow. Any rapid enlargement that occurs other than during pregnancy strongly indicates either degeneration or development of a sarcoma. Growth usually ceases after the menopause. Myomas are named according to their location in the uterus: within the muscle wall, intramural; just below the endometrium, submucous; or encroaching on the outer peritoneal surface of the uterus, subserous. A pedunculated myoma is connected to the uterus by a pedicle and projects into the abdominal cavity (Fig. 7). A fibroid polyp is attached by a pedicle to the uterus within the uterine cavity. Myomas may occur in the cervix, the broad ligament, or may actually become completely detached from the uterus and adhere to adjacent structures (parasitic myomas).

Most myomas are *asymptomatic,* and patients are unaware of their existence until they are quite large. Symptoms, when present, usually occur during the fifth decade of life and occasionally between the ages of 30 and 40 years. Menstrual periods that have increased in amount, duration, and frequency are the most striking symptoms. Continuous flow or spotting more often means malignancy, but if due to myomas, a submucous or polypoid tumor may be present. Other symptoms

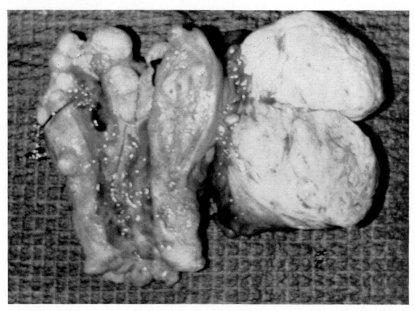

Fig. 7. A large opened pedunculated uterine fibromyoma is shown on the right. In the opened uterus, myomas are seen within the muscle wall (intramural) and immediately beneath the endometrium (submucous).

are unusual, such as pressure or a sense of fullness, since myomas may become very large before any pressure is noted. Pain is *not* a symptom of myoma. If pain is present, additional investigation is necessary. Pain in patients with known myomas usually results from an accident to one of the myomas such as torsion of a pedunculated tumor or degeneration.

Active treatment of myomas is often not indicated since symptoms are not usually present or, if so, are very mild. In most cases surgical therapy may be delayed. Treatment is indicated by the presence and severity of symptoms, the potential danger or risk the patient is subjected to because of tumors, and the presence of coexisting lesions that require treatment. A combination of excessive and prolonged flow frequently indicates the need for treatment. Tumors that are very large in size may possibly degenerate and thus jeopardize the patient's health and life. Pedunculated tumors have a high incidence of torsion, which may result in peritonitis. Therefore, they should be removed. The rapidly growing tumor indicates either degeneration or malignant change and treatment is indicated.

If a patient is being operated upon for some coexisting lesions such as endometriosis, pelvic inflammatory disease, or relaxation lesions, it may be desirable to treat the lesion and the myomas simultaneously.

There are two acceptable methods of management of patients with myomas: (1) nonoperative procedures and (2) operative procedures.

Nonoperative methods are used in all patients who do not require definitive treatment. They are examined every three to six months. Cervical smears for cancer are performed once a year. Slight anemia may be treated by iron and other usual means. Most patients with uterine myomas are treated conservatively, are followed up, and never come to operation.

Operative procedures offer the most satisfactory method of treatment when definitive therapy is indicated. Curettage may suffice as a temporary method of relieving bleeding and excluding the presence of uterine cancer. Myomectomy, removing the myoma but leaving the uterus, is performed on patients who are young and who wish to retain the childbearing function. Hysterectomy, either vaginal or abdominal, is the procedure of choice if there are no contraindications to operations and if the patient's family is complete. This permanently rids the patient of the tumors, obviates further surgical procedures, and removes the hazards of future uterine tumors. The ovaries, unless abnormal, are usually conserved in premenopausal women. They continue to function normally after hysterectomy and therefore should be retained. Women approaching or in the climacteric are usually treated surgically because the abnormal bleeding is more disturbing, the tumors are usually large, and coexisting lesions are more frequently present. In addition, childbearing function is usually completed. Most menopausal patients seldom require treatment for myomas unless abnormal bleeding occurs and/or the tumor continues to grow.

Emotional stresses do arise in some women who are advised to have a hysterectomy or in those who have had a hysterectomy. Prior to operation the patient is reassured that the prime function of the uterus is childbearing and that its removal should have no ill effects on her sense of well-being, sex, or other endocrine functions. It must be emphasized that this is giving an intellectual answer to an emotional subject.

How the woman responds to the experience of hysterectomy is dependent on the significance she places on an intact reproductive tract and the effects she fears it will have on successful marital relations. It is therefore influenced by the wife-husband relationship and by her self-identity as a woman. If she feels that these are threatened by the loss of this organ, even though she knows it is no longer needed for its original function, she may place exceptional emphasis on its removal and loss and on her changed function and self-image. One patient after hysterectomy described herself as "a shell of a woman." With this woman, the stages of grief were clearly observed for a considerable length of time. In some women this response may be lacking (seemingly). Until the patient's life resumes stability and a satisfying structure, she cannot be "told" that the hysterectomy makes her no different. The relationships of the doctor-patient-nurse in the office and hospital during the preoperative and postoperative periods can be beneficial to the patient's postoperative adjustment in teaching her trust, closeness, warmth, concern, and the interdependence of all.

Ovarian tumors. The ovaries are organs in which the potential for neoplastic growth is particularly great. They may contain numerous types of cysts (physiologic, inflammatory, and neoplastic) as well as true tumors.

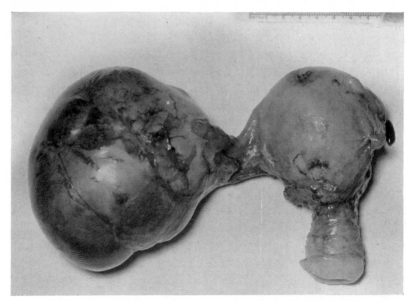

Fig. 8. A "chocolate cyst" of the ovary. It is filled with thick blood that has the appearance of chocolate. The dark areas on the outside of the specimen suggest the presence of endometrial tissue. The corpus and cervix of the uterus were removed with the ovarian cyst.

Retention cysts, follicular and corpus luteum, are usually small and are palpable only occasionally. The patient may have an irregularity of menstrual flow. A rupture of the cyst leading to internal hemorrhage may occasionally occur.

Endometrial cysts are a common manifestation of endometriosis (pp. 105-107). They are usually bilateral, have a tendency to produce dense adhesions, and occur in association with lesions of endometrial tissue or endometriosis throughout the pelvis. They are usually filled with chocolate-colored blood, from which the name "chocolate cyst" has been derived (Fig. 8).

Neoplastic cysts are true tumors. They are named according to their lining epithelium, serous or pseudomucinous, and are filled with either serous or mucinous fluid. They are frequently bilateral and become very large (Fig. 9). Occasionally their lining, instead of being smooth, is covered with papillary processes. These papillary tumors, though histologically benign, are considered potentially malignant and can give rise to carcinoma of the ovary. The *teratoid* or *dermoid tumor* is another neoplastic cyst. These are usually thick-walled and are filled with greasy sebaceous material containing hair and other tissues such as skin, bone, cartilage, and teeth. This tumor has its malignant counterpart, *malignant teratoma,* in which microscopic evidence of several different tissues of the body are seen in their embryonic form. It is one of the most malignant of the ovarian tumors.

Bilateral *polycystic ovaries* are not true tumors but are evidence of some unknown endocrine disturbance. Their occurrence is known as the Stein-Leventhal syndrome and they are characterized by enlarged ovaries, multiple small follicular

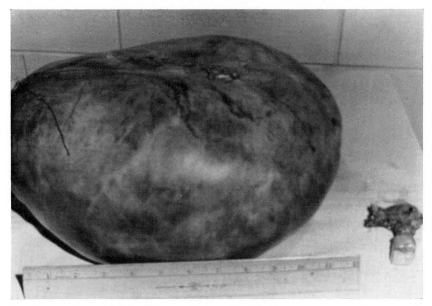

Fig. 9. This ovarian pseudomucinous cyst was completely asymptomatic. Upon questioning, the patient admitted her abdomen seemed to be increasing in size, but she had no other symptoms. The cyst itself weighed approximately 20 pounds. (The uterus and the other tube and ovary were removed at the same time.)

cysts, failure of ovulation, amenorrhea, infertility, and hirsutism. The treatment consists of wedge resection of both ovaries.

Ovarian fibromas are solid benign connective tissue tumors that are usually small and unilateral. They cause no symptoms. Occasionally Meigs' syndrome may be present. This is a benign fibroma of the ovary with ascites and pleural effusion. Removal of the tumor cures the patient.

Brenner tumors are small solid tumors microscopically identified as fibrous tissue stroma interspersed with small masses of epithelium. They are almost always benign.

Functional tumors of the ovary are of two types: (1) feminizing tumors (granulosa and theca-cell) and (2) masculinizing tumors (Leydig cell and others). All are solid tumors and owe their effects to the hormones that they produce. The granulosa and theca-cell tumor effects are due to estrogen. The patient's primary symptoms are abnormal bleeding and the presence of a tumor mass upon examination. The masculinizing tumors are very rare. Their effects are due to secretion of male hormone. The stage of defeminization is followed by masculinization, with hirsutism, changes in the voice, and enlargement of the clitoris. Most of these effects regress when the tumor is removed.

As may be seen, the patient with some kinds of ovarian pathology often has disturbing and fear-provoking physical changes that are apparent to her as well as others. Her disease is often interpreted as strange and distasteful. The teratoid or dermoid tumor and those neoplasms causing changes in feminine character-istics produce this reaction in both patient and nurse. (The doctor, viewing the patient from a different perspective, may describe these entities as "interesting.") The presence of masculinizing characteristics, especially those that may arise as a result of a pathologic condition, is threatening and uncomfortable for most nurses. These patients are frequently avoided and ignored. Regrettably, whether the at-titude of the professions is one of extreme interest in the rare entity or one of withdrawal from its manifestations, the real focus of concern is not on the patient and her emotional reaction to this pathology. She may feel very alone with her abnormality. The attitude of the professions and the ancillary personnel, together with careless bedside discussion, may disturb other patients within the room, and the patient may be further isolated and even ostracized pre- and postoperatively. The environment surrounding this patient can be one of covert and overt hostility unless the nurses recognize the problem and their own feelings and are willing to interpret this for others. They are the only ones who can make the patient's en-vironment a beneficial and therapeutic one for her convalescence.

All ovarian enlargements are treacherous because they may grow quite large, extend, undergo malignant change, and metastasize before any symptoms are present. Symptoms, when present, are often insignificant. The patient may experi-ence abdominal fullness and enlargement or be aware of a mass. Abnormal uterine bleeding may occur; it is usually related to endocrine dysfunction rather than to the tumor itself. Amenorrhea may be associated with follicular and corpus luteum cysts and the hormone-producing solid tumors, followed by abnormal bleeding. Pain as a symptom of an ovarian tumor is usually the result of an accident in the tumor. An accident may be torsion of the tumor pedicle, rupture of an ovarian cyst, hemorrhage into a cyst or from a cyst, and infection.

The differentiation of benign from malignant tumors and physiologic cysts from true neoplastic cysts is determined by the size, shape, consistency, mobility, loca-tion, and reaction of the tumor (tenderness), in addition to associated findings such as fixation and ascites. Tumors that are cystic, under 8 cm. in diameter, and are smooth and freely mobile are most likely physiologic and benign. Solid, fixed, irregular, and bilateral tumors are considered clinically malignant.

Some generalizations can be made concerning the management of ovarian tumors. If a benign physiologic cyst is diagnosed, conservative nonoperative treat-ment may be followed. Small ovarian cysts with no symptoms can often be safely assumed to be physiologic and do not call for surgical intervention. However, it is prudent to reexamine the patient at intervals, since continued growth of the cyst may lead to a change of diagnosis. It is therefore very important that the patient return for recheck examinations. Basically, the treatment of ovarian tumors is sur-gical excision, for this is the only way their actual nature can be determined. If the tumor is benign, it frequently can be resected from the ovary and normal ovarian tissue conserved. Sometimes the ovary involved must be sacrificed, but the other ovary can be preserved.

Pelvic pain

Pelvic pain is a common gynecologic symptom. Because of the multiplicity of etiologic factors, it is difficult to isolate a single cause. Whereas it is frequently engendered in the reproductive tract, it may also originate in the gastrointestinal or urinary tracts, bones, joints, muscles, or nerves. Psychogenic causes must also be considered.

A history may frequently determine the source of pain. If the onset follows abortion, cautery, or instrumentation, a streptococcal pelvic infection is probable. If it is associated with amenorrhea, a complication of pregnancy must be considered. If it is associated with stooping, bending, or lifting, bones, joints, muscles, or nerves may be the source. Sudden onset may mean an acute, serious condition such as an intraperitoneal hemorrhage. Severe bilateral lower abdominal pain associated with fever and cervical and adnexal tenderness means acute inflammatory disease. Acquired dysmenorrhea and dyspareunia are indicative of endometriosis.

Colicky, cramping pain usually means a hollow viscus is involved. Abortion, tubal pregnancy, organic and functional bowel problems, intestinal obstruction, ureteral stones, or congenital reproductive system anomalies may be associated with cramping pain. Pain aggravated by defecation may indicate rectal endometriosis, malignancy, or infection.

Radiation of pain to the legs and back is more often urinary tract than genital in origin, but it may be secondary to pelvic malignancy or infection. Many painful conditions are associated with tumors that may or may not be apparent on examination. These too must be considered.

Accurate diagnosis is often dependent on the ability and willingness of the patient to communicate her pain (Chapter 2).

Endometriosis. Endometriosis is a benign lesion in which endometrial tissue is found in various ectopic locations. The lesions are usually found in the pelvis, but on rare occasion they may be found elsewhere in the body. Endometriosis is more prevalent in private than in clinic patients. It often coexists with myomas in white patients, but is rarely encountered in Negroes. There are several theories of the histogenesis of endometriosis. The most common explanations are that endometrial tissue is transported to ectopic sites through the uterine tubes by a retrograde flow during menstruation, it is transported by mechanical instrumentation during an operative procedure, or it is transported by lymphatic or venous spread. Endometriosis may develop in ectopic locations as a result of metaplasia. It may occur due to direct extension through the myometrium. It may develop through a combination of several of these mechanisms. External endometriosis refers to all lesions of endometrial tissue outside the uterus. Internal endometriosis (adenomyosis) specifies endometrial tissue located deep in the uterine wall.

Acquired dysmenorrhea developing in a woman between 20 and 35 years of age is very suggestive of endometriosis. Acquired progressive dyspareunia is another common symptom. Sterility and abnormal uterine bleeding may also occur, although both of these symptoms may be incidental complaints. Frequently the symptoms in no way reflect the extent of the lesion. Those with few symptoms may have extensive disease and those with severe complaints may have minimal lesions.

Fixed tender nodules in the region of the uterosacral ligaments and fixed tender ovarian cysts are the most characteristic findings upon bimanual examination. The uterus may also be restricted in motion due to dense adhesions, which are characteristic of endometriosis. Vaginal and cervical lesions may be seen.

At operation, typical small, blue-black, or brown puckered lesions may be seen on the peritoneal surfaces of the bladder, uterus, ovaries, cul-de-sac, uterosacral ligaments, and rectum. The histologic diagnosis depends on microscopic identification of the endometrial glands and stroma. Since small lesions may be missed at the time of pathologic study, the designation "endometriosis, surgical diagnosis" is added to the patient's record.

Surgical treatment is indicated only in those patients with symptoms that interfere with health or function. Symptoms moderately severe can often be alleviated by nonsurgical means. In patients approaching the climacteric the lesions may be expected to regress with the termination of menstruation. In younger patients childbearing may proceed before operative treatment becomes necessary.

Medical management consists of the administration of hormones that block ovulation and thus alleviate the prime symptom of dysmenorrhea. Relief of symptoms with either estrogen or progesterone or both may be expected in 70 to 80% of the patients. It may be possible to forestall an operation for a considerable length of time.

Conservative surgical procedures are indicated for severe and extensive disease when the childbearing function is to be conserved. The objective of the conservative surgical procedure is toward the relief of symptoms and the removal of interference with childbearing. Resection of ovarian endometrial cysts, other endometriotic implants, and lysis of adhesions are the procedures of choice. Every effort is made to preserve childbearing function in a woman under 35 years of age whose family is not complete, knowing that there may be a 25% recurrence rate of endometriosis requiring operation. The fertility rate subsequent to such conservative operations varies, with the reported average being approximately 30%.

Frequently it is not possible to determine prior to operation whether a conservative or radical procedure may be required. In women 35 to 45 years old, ovarian tissue is saved if possible; after 45 years of age the more radical procedure predominates. Total hysterectomy will usually alleviate most of the symptoms of this disease, and it is not always necessary to remove the ovaries, although ovarian secretions are necessary for the lesions to grow. Lesions in the intestine and urinary bladder are resected if possible. However, when lesions occur in the intestine, bladder lumen, or ureteral regions, the operative procedure is a bilateral oophorectomy, which results in a prompt regression of lesions. Individualization of patients is essential, and many exceptions are made. The treatment given is based on the symptoms, findings, and the desire for children. Conservation is observed whenever possible.

Ovulation and menstruation cease with the bilateral removal of the ovaries. The patient is said to have a surgical menopause; that is, menses cease due to the operation and she enters the climacteric period of her life. Younger patients fear the effect of this on their sexual experience and also the effect of physical changes such as skin texture, emotional changes, weight gain, and increased susceptibility to coronary artery disease. The latter is a worry to many women facing bilateral oophorectomy. Many lay articles in magazines and newspapers have aroused this worry. These patients are usually started on early hormone therapy. This alleviates the effects of sudden hormone withdrawal and eliminates some of the feared sequelae of the operation. Further discussion of the symptoms and changes during the climacteric are to be found on pp. 114-116.

Adenomyosis. Adenomyosis is a condition in which islands of endometrium are located within the uterine wall. Its primary symptom is abnormal uterine bleeding in women over 35 years of age. This may be persistent, excessive, and prolonged menstrual flow and may be associated with dysmenorrhea. Physical examination reveals a symetrically enlarged and firm uterus. Treatment depends upon the severity of the bleeding and pain. Hysterectomy is the treatment of choice.

Pelvic inflammatory disease. By common usage in some hospitals, P.I.D. or pelvic inflammatory disease is used as a synonym of venereal disease. This is not correct. The patient with pelvic inflammatory disease is systemically ill, usually with a high fever. She experiences extreme pelvic tenderness. This is particularly evident during examination when the cervix is moved. Gonorrhea, one of the entities associated with pelvic inflammatory disease, is also a venereal disease. The other common etiologic agents of pelvic inflammatory disease—*Streptococcus, Staphylococcus,* and *Mycobacterium tuberculosis*—are not associated with venereal transmission.

Gonorrhea. The patient's first and only symptoms may be a yellowish discharge and burning and frequency of urination. This may soon subside and the incident is forgotten. During the initial progression of the disease the paraurethral glands (Skene's) and ducts are frequently involved, as well as Bartholin's glands. This results in urethritis and/or abscess of Skene's and Bartholin's glands.

When a Bartholin infection has progressed to abscess formation, there is severe pain, local redness, and swelling. It is often too painful for the patient to sit or to walk. Spontaneous rupture may occur or an incision and drainage of the abscess may be performed. Symptomatic cysts may be excised. Later in the disease the organism involves the cervix, endometrium, and ultimately the uterine tubes, causing gonorrheal salpingitis. Both tubes are usually infected, which frequently results in tubal closure and sterility. There may be pyosalpinx ("pus tubes"), followed by hydrosalpinx, pelvic adhesions, or tubo-ovarian masses.

Penicillin is still the antibiotic of choice in the treatment of acute salpingitis due to gonorrhea. If treated promptly and adequately, the sequela of gonorrhea frequently do not occur. The residues of salpingitis, so-called chronic salpingitis, may cause no symptoms, although large tubo-ovarian masses and adhesions are present. Symptoms, when present, are pain, bleeding, and sterility. The treatment of these residues is dependent on the symptoms. Usually treatment is nonsurgical except in those patients who have severe pain or bleeding. Occasionally the tubes are closed at the fimbriated ends only. The possibility of successful tuboplasty does exist, although infrequently.

Tuberculosis. Genital tuberculosis is usually secondary to a lesion elsewhere in the body, such as the lungs, urinary tract, bowel, or bone. The diagnosis is suggested in patients not responding to the usual treatment for tuberculosis diagnosed elsewhere in the body. Genital tuberculosis also is suspected in the patient who has an infertility problem. Tuberculin tests and chest and kidney x-ray examinations help in making the diagnosis. The actual diagnosis may be made by finding the organisms in smears and cultures from the vaginal secretions, from collection of menstrual flow, from endometrial biopsies, and from curettage.

In early cases of genital tuberculosis, medical treatment with streptomycin, para-aminosalicylic acid, and isonicotinic acid hydrazide are proving successful. Unfortunately, in more advanced tuberculosis, pain, bleeding, inflammatory masses, and adhesions are so great that medical therapy has little curative value. The uterine tubes, endometrium, pelvic peritoneum, and cervix may be involved. The best treatment then is surgical removal.

Streptococcal and staphylococcal infections. Pelvic inflammatory disease of streptococcal or staphylococcal origin is usually the result of trauma to the genital tract. The trauma may be post instrumentation, such as cautery, radium, criminal abortion, or operative and obstetric procedures. Large doses of the specific antibiotic are given.

Leukorrhea

A normal clear mucus vaginal secretion is almost always present in the female. All other blood-free vaginal discharges are known as leukorrhea and are indicative of an abnormal process. Leukorrhea is probably the most common of all gynecologic symptoms. It may forewarn of tumors of the genital tract such as polyps and carcinoma. However, the more common causes of leukorrhea are vaginitis and cervicitis.

Vaginitis. Vaginitis may be caused by the organisms of *Candida albicans, Trichomonas vaginalis,* or *Haemophilus vaginalis;* it may be due to a foreign body reaction or a nonspecific infection. These are the most frequent vaginal infections. Vaginitis is characterized by leukorrhea and itching. The vaginal mucous membranes and often the vulva are red and show evidence of scratching. The diagnosis is made by microscopic examination of a wet mount. A bit of material obtained from the vagina with a speculum is placed on a slide in a warm drop of saline solution, covered with a cover slip, and then studied under the microscope. Cultures may also be made.

Mycotic vulvovaginitis (Candida albicans) is characterized by a thick white discharge in which mycelial forms or the budding forms of yeast may be identified.

The vaginitis caused by *Trichomonas vaginalis* is characterized by a thin white frothy discharge which is profuse. Microscopic examination of the discharge reveals a typical pear-shaped mobile flagellate.

The vaginitis resulting from *Haemophilus vaginalis* is characterized by a foul odor; the discharge may vary in color from white or gray to yellow and may vary in consistency from thin to curdy. The wet mount shows characteristic "clue cells" which are large vaginal epithelial cells with a very granular cytoplasm and an indefinite membrane. There are usually very few leukocytes in the smear.

The diagnosis of nonspecific vaginitis is made only after ruling out the other forms of vaginitis and gonococcal infections. Microscopically, leukocytes and bacteria are seen.

There are specific forms of therapy for each of the different types of vaginitis. Medication is administered orally or by douche or suppository. These infections may be very difficult to eradicate and treatment may be long and disappointing. The course of therapy is extended through the period of menses if it occurs during the span of administration. Pruritus is often severe, especially at night (Chapter 2).

The nurse can extend help to these patients until the therapy is effective. She can explain the factors that inhibit and enhance itching. The patient may then feel a participant in her own recovery by avoiding those factors that stimulate pruritus. She can decrease the pruritus experience, feel greater confidence in the therapy, and derive greater therapeutic benefit from the medication. These patients often need someone with whom they can confide their miserable discomfort.

Leukorrhea is troublesome and embarrassing to a woman. Many fastidious women even complain about the normal vaginal secretions and are accustomed to daily or periodic douching. (This is inadvisable.) When leukorrhea exists, the soiling of undergarments, pruritus, and often a foul odor provoke anxieties about genital infection, a subject that is taboo. Patients most frequently worry about *how* they *acquired* the vaginitis and *why*. The young unmarried woman experiences dread and shame at the time of her first visit to the doctor. The married woman, too, worries about how and why she acquired the infection and whether she will infect her husband.

The organisms responsible for vaginitis are often found in the normal vaginal flora. They produce inflammatory vaginitis when the pH of the secretion changes or a changed internal environment of the patient enhances their rapid reproduction. For example, systemic changes in the diabetic patient or prolonged antibiotic therapy often permits the development of *Candida albicans*. This should be explained to patients physically suffering from vaginitis who also emotionally are suffering the fear of censure by doctor or nurse because of the presence of the infection itself.

The patient's husband usually is asymptomatic, though the organisms may be present in the genital organ. Unless therapy is also initiated for him, the patient may have a recurrent infection after her therapy is discontinued. During the course of medication therapy, sexual relations are avoided. The douche tip, can, or bag should be kept clean between use and it should be used by only one person. *All equipment should be sterilized before use by another.*

Cervicitis. Cervicitis is the second most frequent cause of leukorrhea. It is an inflammation involving the ectocervix, endocervix, or both. The discharge is thick and mucopurulent. The cervix appears red and granular. This must be differentiated from cancer of the cervix. Therefore, it is very important that a complete investigation for cervical carcinoma be made. This includes vaginal smears and cervical biopsies. Following negative reports, the diagnosis may then be considered cervicitis and the cervix may be cauterized by electric cautery. The patient is requested to return four to seven days after menses has ceased. Cauterization may be done in the office, since the cervix is relatively free of pain fibers. When pain *is* experienced by the patient, it is not the sharp stinging pain associated with a burn, but deep aching pain which is usually located in the low back or thighs (Chapter 2).

Probably most disturbing to the patient are her unique thoughts and images associated with burning tissue, especially *within* an orifice. It is also disturbing that her anticipation of when the pain will occur and the quality of the pain are different from the actual experience. Initially, the patient is often only aware of the tactile sensation of the inserted speculum, the auditory clue of the crackling electricity of the cautery tip, and *infrequently* a thermal sensation of warmth. The olfactory stimulus that is correctly interpreted as burning tissue and the realization that this is *her* "burning flesh" is often her first proof that the cauterization actually is being performed. These combined sensations and the realization of burning may provoke mounting apprehension in the patient. Pain, nausea, perspiration, increased pulse and respirations, and faintness (or actual syncope) emphasize the emotional stress to the patient.

The establishment of close doctor-patient and nurse-patient relationships *before* the procedure, which are maintained *throughout* the procedure by sincere understanding and open communication, help the patient to retain confidence and trust in the therapy and the doctor and to be assured of the understanding and goodwill of those helping her. Her anxiety will be minimal, if it exists at all, within such an interpersonal environment. This can be a therapeutically beneficial environment that augments the healing expectations of the therapy. After cauterization the patient may expect some abnormal bleeding as well as an actual increase in leukorrhea for a few weeks. The patient should be examined every month for several months in order that the doctor may determine and/or prevent a cervical stricture.

Venereal disease

The group of diseases that are transmitted by sexual intercourse are known as venereal diseases. They are becoming an alarming health problem, rapidly increasing all over the world. There is a particularly rapid increase in the incidence of venereal disease among adolescents in America within the past few years. Syphilis, gonorrhea, lymphopathia venereum, granuloma inguinale, and chancroid are venereal diseases. The initial lesions may be located in the genitalia. However, in syphilis the initial lesion may involve skin or mucous membranes other than genital. The diversified symptoms and the nongynecologic ramifications of the total disease cannot be discussed within the scope of this book. Sources for this information are suggested in the suggested readings at the end of the chapter.

With modern methods of treatment, the majority of patients are noninfectious soon after therapy has begun. The risk of accidental infection of the nurse and other paramedical personnel is slight or absent. These patients, if admitted to a hospital, are placed within the general medical units and are not isolated. Therapy usually is given through the clinic or office.

Ignorance, in combination with a relaxed moral code, is the one great single factor in the spread of venereal disease. Explanation of the risks and dangers involved in the infections, prevention, and treatment are prime objectives of public education. Disregard for and contempt for the so-called health hazards occasioned by the venereal diseases arose during the early era of penicillin when infection rates were high but treatment was easy, quick, and sure. Succeeding generations have seen few examples of tertiary syphilis or congenital syphilis. Greater mobility of people, decreased family identification, fluctuating moral codes, social instability, and world tensions have been identified as important factors in the increase of these diseases. Social or marital problems frequently lead to the initial infection and to repeated infections. The social service department of the hospital or clinic is of exceptional help to these patients, extending personal and family counseling, with psychologic and psychiatric referral when needed. The school nurse or a referral from her often provides this to the adolescent.

As with all infections involving the reproductive organs, nonvenereal and venereal, shame, guilt, and therefore delay in seeking help are usual. This is a costly delay to the future of the patient. The availability of the helping professions to the patient is a determining factor. It is difficult and sometimes impossible to ask help of someone who looks down on the one seeking help or of someone who judges and sentences the individual seeking help. It is also difficult for the patient to seek help from one who expects the rewards of his fellowman because he has associated with and given to one whose predicament is lower than his own. These generalities are presented as guides.

Patients with infection of the genital tract present one main challenge to the helping professions: the establishment of a true empathic relationship. When concern for the individual exists, combined with goodwill for her and respect for her potential as an individual regardless of her current state, two individuals will try to understand one another, to openly communicate, and to give and receive. When one member of the relationship is a patient, her need to receive is greater than her ability to give; even her ability to "give" communicative expression is hindered. The one capable of helping, either physically, emotionally, or intellectually, is the member of a helping-healing profession. If she feels that the recipient (patient) is unworthy of her giving, she will withhold or give stintingly. If she gives because her religion, profession, or family code says she should, then her giving will assuage their demands of her, but the true needs of the patient may never be evaluated. It is for this reason that mandates cannot be given when personal relationships are involved. It is futile to say, "The nurse must be kind, considerate, understanding, nonjudgmental, etc." If given because of such orders, the attempted kindness, consideration, or understanding are shams of sincerity.

It is only when an individual is willing to trust another, to be open and put aside her mask that hides who she really is, that she can respond with kindness and consideration to another and can begin to understand an individual different from and yet like herself. The instigation of therapy, the continuation of therapy, and the prevention of venereal disease itself is dependent on the quality of such relationships between the patient and the helping-healing professions and the patient and her community. Sometimes the nurse is the bridge between the two.

Sterility

In the majority of patients who do not conceive there is no absolute sterility in either marital partner, but rather a relative infertility brought about by a multiplicity of factors in both partners. These are usually insufficient to cause infertility in themselves, but in combination they may prevent conception. Thus a more accurate term than "sterility" would be "barren marriage" since this emphasizes the mutual liabilities of both husband and wife in the wife's failure to conceive.

Success in the relief of a barren marriage demands adequate examination of both the husband and the wife, followed by systematic elimination of all contributing factors. This may require the assistance of a urologist, internist, and/or an endocrinologist. Since it is usually the gynecologist who is consulted first in such problems, he is obligated to discover the factors that contribute to the infertility. His examination includes the general history and physical survey, the study of the uterine cervix and its secretions, a testing of the uterine tubes for patency, an investigation of the endocrine system, and an analysis of the man's semen. A general physical examination and a genital examination of both partners are obtained.

The actual survey of the infertile couple begins with the semen analysis. This is because 40 to 50% of all infertility problems are due to the man. Many elaborate, time-consuming, and expensive studies of the woman can be avoided if absolute sterility is found in the man. If any abnormality of the sperm is found, the husband is referred to a urologist.

Evaluation of the woman for an ovulation profile must be obtained. She is instructed to take her basal body temperature each morning before arising. The typical basal temperature chart of a patient who is ovulating and menstruating regularly (approximately every 28 days) shows a low temperature on the twelfth day and sustained elevated temperatures from the fourteenth through the twenty-seventh days. Other commonly used tests for the presence of ovulation are vaginal

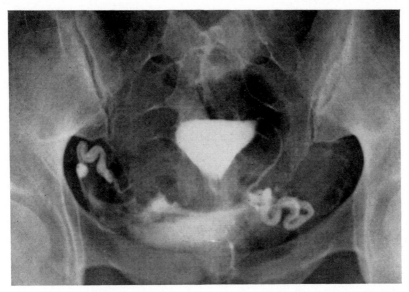

Fig. 10. A normal uterosalpingogram, showing contrast media in the uterus and in both tubes, with bilateral intraperitoneal spill. This indicates that both uterine tubes are patent.

smears, studies of the cervical mucus, and endometrial biopsy. Cervical mucus, when dried on an ordinary glass slide, shows a definite fernlike crystallization pattern during the first half of the menstrual cycle under the influence of estrogen. If the patient ovulates, this ferning will be inhibited by progesterone and in the second half of the menstrual cycle this pattern will not be present. An endometrial biopsy showing a secretory type of endometrium indicates ovulation. Tubal patency tests are done by inserting carbon dioxide in special instruments through the uterine tubes or by injecting a radiopaque media into the uterus and through the tubes and taking an x-ray film (Fig. 10).

While the examination procedure was initiated to include both partners, the extensiveness and prolonged testing of the woman tends to emphasize to her that *she is* at fault. Thus the psychologic reaction of the patient to the many examinations and the time involved must be evaluated. Many nationalities still emphasize the selection of a wife who possesses apparent qualities of fertility and ease of childbearing. The childless couple from such background has the family's censure to cope with in addition to their own individual feelings. To many family units the adoption of another's child is not a substitute and is not acceptable as a continuation of the lineal heritage. To some families the family line seems to be little considered. Whether the pressure of this factor is felt or not, the individual failure of the woman to procreate is felt deeply by both wife and husband. One more pressure is brought to bear on them. Large families and early families are rather commonplace today. Thus even the current societal trend places certain expectations on the married couple. Their peers look askance when they do not conform. The husband's virility and the wife's femininity are questioned.

Hospital nurses seldom know the patient with this problem; that is, they seldom know her as a gynecologic patient. Often she may be a patient hospitalized for other causes who also bears the unresolved problem of infertility. The hospital nurse or the industrial, clinic, office, or public health nurse learns of these problems when the patient feels safe with her, when she feels comfortable in her presence, and when she feels confident in her ability to help her. The quality of the nurse-patient relationship determines the patient's request for help and the amount of help she will accept. Preceding her referral to the doctor and as an adjunct to his counseling, the nurse, as an understanding professional woman, can extend the help needed.

Treatment of the woman depends on improving her general health as well as correction of any abnormal genital factors (cervical, uterine, tubal, or ovarian). Uterine retroversion, hyperplasia, and fibroids rarely are factors involved in infertility. Vaginitis and cervicitis, if present, are treated. Infertility due to tubal occlusion is becoming less frequent with antibiotic treatment of gonorrhea and tuberculosis. Surgical correction of tubal closure is still unsatisfactory, with less than 13% successful pregnancies following tuboplastic procedures. In addition, there is a high incidence of tubal pregnancies following these operations.

The treatment of the failure to ovulate depends on the accurate diagnosis of the problem. Ovarian resection will be most successful for the patient with polycystic ovaries. Therapy with estrogens, progesterones, and other hormones, as advocated by many clinicians, have been most disappointing in the production of ovulation. New drugs (chlomiphene and Pergonal) now being used experimentally have given great promise in stimulating ovulation. In patients with adrenal dysfunction (adrenal-genital syndrome) cortisone is the treatment of choice and is very successful.

Occasionally the diagnostic survey itself may be therapeutic, since a number of patients will conceive following patency tests. The psychologic aspects of infertility have been widely discussed and certainly play a role involving both partners. This is particularly true when a change of climate or occupation, vacations, or adoptions have been followed by pregnancy.

CLIMACTERIC PERIOD

The woman in the United States today often has at least most of her family reared and off to work or college by the time she is 40 to 45 years old. This means that childbearing and care of the very young child do not extend throughout the full span of the childbearing years. Rather, this phase is focused on the early years of her marriage. This is an important factor to consider in the woman as she approaches the climacteric period of her life.

To the extent she has achieved satisfactions in her maternal role of nurture to a young dependent family, she becomes increasingly able to develop a maturing role to her family as she helps them to grow and achieve varying stages of independence from her. Her ultimate goal is the fulfillment of a new family unit, a new generation, in which her role is one of providing continuity and guidance to the lineal line. This assumes her ability to change roles, to be willing to accept the independence of her children, to master interdependent relationships with them, and to so reconstruct her life that it will retain purpose, direction, and satisfactions.

The woman who has been unwilling or unable to adjust to changes in the extent of her responsibilities, to the changes in her relationship with her husband and the growing family, to the changes in herself and the children, and to the realization that she is not needed in the same way anymore will be abruptly faced with many physical, emotional, and social adjustments within the transition period—the climacteric. It is toward an identification of these problems and their solution that many women in the climacteric period seek help. These are the recurrent themes in their conversation as they talk with the doctor and nurse.

The woman should also anticipate and recognize physical changes occurring in her. At 30 years of age she does not expect to engage in the intense activities of the 18-year-old. In the years of premenarche she was gradually prepared by visual signs and thoughtful counseling for the physical and emotional changes that occurred with the onset of the menarche and the adolescent years of transition. So the young mature woman should gradually prepare for continuing changes in her physical and emotional life, even as she changes her goals, her expectations, and her tastes. The climacteric period is a normal period of life during which the reproductive ability of the woman gradually ceases. The physiologic changes can be affected by the personal philosophy of the woman toward her life, her fear and distrust of the future, and the pressures of her environment upon her.

The climacteric period is the normal and physiologic termination of the reproductive phase of the woman's life. Women who enjoy good general health maintain their freshness and "well-being" for years. This "well-being" is frequently enhanced by the physical relief from the recurring discomforts of the menstrual cycle and the removal of the fear of pregnancy. Eighty percent of women pass though this period with no ill effects whatsoever. In most of the other 20% the symptoms are mild. Even with severe symptoms, a woman can be assured relatively easy relief.

Some changes do take place. The ovaries cease to ovulate, but they continue to secrete female hormone—estrogen. The uterus, tubes, and ovaries do become smaller and atrophic over a period of years. The vaginal changes, which usually occur several years after the menopause, consist of atrophy of the epithelial lining. The breasts also atrophy. Essentially, there is no change in other glands. The main symptom of the menopause is cessation of menses. Usually there is a gradual disappearance, with the flow becoming scanty, of shorter duration, and less frequent. An increased flow or decreased interval is indicative of pelvic disease. The other symptoms of the period are based on vasomotor instability. These are the so-called hot flushes and flashes, sweats, and emotional problems.

For generations this period has falsely been considered a critical period because of the fear of mental instability. No permanent psychic changes occur in normal women *as a result* of the climacteric.

The effect on the libido or the sex drive is variable. In the majority of women there is no change. A happy and compatible sex life with a considerate and understanding husband will continue unchanged. A few women have decreased libido and, on the other hand, some have a definite increase.

A very small minority of patients have severe enough symptoms to require treatment. Usually sedatives and reassurance suffice. If not, simple, cheap, and efficient methods of treatment are available due to the development of oral hormone therapy. Hypodermic injections of female sex hormone are not necessary over a prolonged period of time. They are uncomfortable, expensive, and no more effective than the oral medication. Occasionally they are used when quick relief is desired, and this is then followed by oral hormone therapy.

If this period is actually a critical period, it is because of the increased incidence of physical problems in this age group—benign or malignant tumors, cardiovascular-renal disease, and diabetes. Periodic medical checkups continue to be necessary, even though the woman has ceased to menstruate.

It is to be emphasized that the current time span of a woman's life after the menopause is often as long as (or longer than) the entire childbearing period. She may have a 30 to 35 year life span after the cessation of menses. Unless maturation and stable relationships have occurred prior to this time, the climacteric and the years beyond are often wrought with days of tension, emotional distress, and depression.

The nurse requires a knowledge of her own feelings about the changing and maturing roles of a woman. If she thinks of life as a continuum of activity, function, and responsibility, she will be able to help a patient prepare for and assume new roles and responsibilities as her personal environment changes. She requires a new purpose for her giving within different periods of her life. If the nurse is clinging to the youthful era of life and is apprehensive or unappreciative of later maturity, she will be unable to help the climacteric woman. She may be impatient because of the patient's fears of purposelessness and lack of direction. She will not recognize the emotional and physical stresses of this transition period. She may pity her and, by so devaluing her abilities and potentials, she may be unable to see any plan for her life or any hope for her future. Students or nurses of any age who are unaware of their own feelings of life, work, sickness, and death can help patients only on a superficial plane. Self-knowledge is basic to an understanding of others, respecting others, or "supporting" others. Office nurses who are sought by the troubled climacteric woman know that much of the time spent by them is ineffectual to the patient because they try to solve the problems, they cannot listen, or because they become uncomfortable and even engender hostile feelings. These are often correctly interpreted by the patient; yet in her extreme need to find herself, the woman seeks the help of this professional woman. The climacteric patient provides the greatest challenge to the nurse for optimum interviewing and counseling skills.

RECOMMENDED READINGS FOR INSTRUCTORS

Brewer, John I.: Textbook of gynecology. Baltimore, 1961, The Williams & Wilkins Co.

Catterall, R. D.: Venerology for nurses, A textbook of the sexually transmitted diseases, London, 1964, English Universities Press, Ltd.

Cohen, M. R.: A simplified plan for the infertile couple, Postgraduate Medicine **36:**337-342, 1964.

Sheets, J. L., Symmonds, R. E., and Banner, E. A.: Conservative surgical management of endometriosis, Obstetrics and Gynecology **23:**625-628, 1964.

The woman in America, Daedalus, Spring, 1964. (Contributors: Lotte Bailyn, Jill Conway, Carl Degler, Erik Erikson, Joan Erikson, Esther Peterson, David Riesman, Alice Rossi, and Edna Rostow.)

TYPICAL READINGS ACCESSIBLE TO PATIENTS

Anderson, Kenneth N.: Is the pill the answer? Today's Health **43**(16):28-34, 70, 1965.

Lake, Alice: Menopause, is it necessary? Good Housekeeping **160**(4):85, 158, 160, 162, 164, 1965.

Ogg, Elizabeth: A new chapter in family planning, Public Affairs Pamphlet No. 1360, Washington, 1964, Public Affairs Press.

Robbins, Jhan, and Robbins, June: Those new fertility drugs, Good Housekeeping **160**(3): 88, 197-200, 1965.

Chapter 7

The postclimacteric patient

How is "old" defined? By a child and adolescent it may be defined as any individual older than they; by the third generation, a grandparent or gray hair; by young parents in their twenties, anyone who has reared a family or a woman after the menopause. By those of later ages it may be defined as retirement age or a chronologic age that is set later and later, depending on the age of the evaluator; by the working class, physical decline after physical prime; by the upper class, accumulated knowledge, wisdom, or acknowledged social standing. The sociologist may describe "old" as a change in social function or the legal age set by the Federal Social Security Act: 65 years for men, 62 years for women. To the psychologist it means changes in perception and mental acuity objectively measured as changes in vision, hearing, and memory and subjectively measured as "you're as old as you feel." The biologist thinks of it in terms of evidences of progressive wearing out and degenerative tissue changes such as the "aging" thymus gland in the infant, the continuously "aging" red blood cells, the "aging" female reproductive organs, or degenerative vascular changes, especially in the kidney, heart, and brain.

Who is the climacteric woman? Functionally, she is the woman who has lost her function of childbearing. Biologically, she has had involutional changes in the reproductive organs, with decreased hormonal secretion, cessation of menstruation (menopause), changes in skin texture, and vascular changes. Sometimes the latter produces symptoms of flushing, perspiration, or headaches. The climacteric period ends when these symptoms abate.

THE OLDER PATIENT AND THE NURSE

The most damaging influence on the older woman and those approaching old age is the prevailing attitude of the society surrounding them. Our age has been called the "Century of the Child,"* with an overemphasis of youthful goals. Its values are those of vitality, newness, mobility, and change. Age is considered generally unattractive and unrewarding. This feeling is reinforced by evidences of the loneliness and isolation of the aged, their lack of independence, their loss of physical attractiveness and prestige, and their diminishing goals of the future.* Death may be reality for all ages, but for the aged it is part of the present. *"Non*-being is hard to grasp while we are *in*-being. . . . Our society, which is oriented toward 'being' and 'doing,' has little sympathy for 'non-being' and 'non-doing.' "†

Rejection may be reflected in the form of hostility, impatience, or sentimentality. Subjected to the feelings of society, which were often fostered and nourished by the individual herself as a younger woman, the older woman may experience self-depreciation. If the adolescent is seeking to attain self-identity and recognition in a mature society and a mature individual is seeking to *maintain* this within the society, then the older individual may be considered to be striving to *retain* self-identity and recognition.

The distance of years and interests, uneasiness in the presence of adult dependency, and anger or frustration toward society's treatment of the aged contribute to the misunderstandings and apprehensions that exist between the generations.

It should not be surprising that student nurses in our society also have definite feelings about the older patient, despite their altruistic goals of patient care. Student nurses have commented, "It's hard when they're patients in the hospital. It's really hard for a young nurse to get *down* to their level and to reassure an 80-year-old woman. Our interests are so different and you don't know what to say. We don't have many older nurses. Sometimes if there's another older patient, they can console one another."

The student nurse or young gradute nurse feels inadequacies in herself when she is required to counsel, comfort, or teach those who may be of her grandparents' generation or older. In the older patient's presence the young nurse may actually experience the feelings of being the grandchild. Without the perceptive understanding and guidance of her instructor or head nurse, she may feel uncomfortable and inadequate to assume a surrogate mother role to a woman of this generation. She may find it difficult to bathe and "feed" and "give" to the extent that she once received from them. Self-conscious hands are often clumsy and rough; impatience and uneasiness with self are often directed to the person who initiates or magnifies the feeling.

The nurse is particularly involved in the dilemma of how to help the elderly patient. If she rushes in to do for the "vulnerable" and "helpless," she also knows

---

*Lukas, Edwin, quoted in Linden, Maurice E.: Relationship between social attitudes toward aging and the delinquencies of youth, American Journal of Psychiatry **114:**444, 1957.

†Lowy, Louis: Social group work with older people. Proceedings of a seminar held at Lake Mohonk, New Paltz, N. Y., June 5-10, 1961, National Association of Social Workers, p. 50.

it is "good" to help the patient help herself. *How much* and *how* the nurse helps are really controlled by *why* she helps. Does she help the elderly patient because her slowness or diminished dexterity makes it easier and quicker for the nurse to do it? Does she help the patient because she feels sorry for her? Does she help the patient in order to see the results of her efforts? Does she allow the patient to take care of herself because the patient's demands are difficult for her to tolerate?

The patient is accorded an inferior place and is in a helpless state when a nurse decides that she would not understand, cannot help, or is not able to cope with the situation. Contact with older patients arouses the following student responses:

> She wanted to be generally cooperative, but she doesn't know how to go about it. She hinders things more than she helps. Right before they took her down for a curettage, they took her to the gynecologic examination room for an examination. She wanted to help by getting up on the cart herself. It's much easier for an older patient to slide from the bed to the cart. But she said, "No, no, dear. I'll get up there myself. You don't have to help me." She stumbled and she tried to help but she hindered things even more. Even if she isn't succeeding, she is trying, and I guess you have to give her credit for that.

> They take so much longer. Everything is geared to a slower degree. She didn't want to be real fussy, but she just naturally was that way. A lot of patients don't realize that you have a lot of other things to do and other patients to take care of. I don't think she really knew how busy the ward was that morning.

> He's [the doctor] busy you know, but she wouldn't let him go on with his rounds. She went right down her list of questions and then sometimes she couldn't remember her notes. She wanted to know about the x-rays, if she still had to take her vitamin pills, and if she would return to the clinic, and she wanted to tell him about the pain she had when she voided. He usually is able to spend only two or three minutes with each patient because he goes around to see them all, but she had this big list of questions.

These patients were attempting to control their diminishing sphere of participation and to control some aspect of self-direction. That their attempt and motive were unsuccessful may be assumed from the condescension shown and the censure present in the narration of the incidents. One wonders did these patients ever try again, or did they give up? Can the need for help be anticipated by the professions and help extended *before* the time of crucial need? If so, the patient would not experience this later defeat, helplessness, and dependence and the resulting humiliation and frustration.

To anticipate the need for help requires perception and sensitivity to the individual and her existing environment. To extend the kind and amount of help that will best assist each patient requires fortitude to act. It also requires personal insight and integrity to recognize that unselfish help extended *before* emergency situations arise often is unrecognized by the patient or others. It involves giving freely in optimum measure *without* the rewards of gratitude or recognition.

The nurse therefore must be aware of the physical changes that necessitate help of others. Certain physical changes may or may not be present in the older patient. Their presence does not always mean a change in function or disability, nor are physical changes to be related to chronologic age. However, recognition and evaluation of the changes and their combined influence on other functions influence nursing of the aging gynecologic patient.

For example, an elderly patient with skeletal changes may find the examining table an extremely hard obstacle course. She may find it difficult to step up backward and she may attempt to sit down on a table higher than she estimates. If the patient also has a diminution of kinesthetic sense and/or visual perception, the task is almost impossible without accident if unassisted. An elderly patient may feel more secure getting onto the table by using a footstool, which affords her more ease of movement and sense of security. If the step end of the table is used, she may require firm physical support to supplement diminished muscle power. Decreased cardiac output may make a perfectly flat position on the table very uncomfortable for her. Decreased proprioception and knee joint stiffness may combine to confound the patient trying to find the stirrups. A combination of all these obstacles, a feeling of time pressure for undressing and preparing for the examination, plus the reason for the examination itself may produce an anxious and harried patient before the examination even begins.

Decreased vaginal secretions and aging tissue changes make the pelvic examination of the older patient *more uncomfortable* than for a younger one. It is necessary for the nurse to understand this. Optimum relaxation of the patient is necessary. This will be dependent on her preliminary preparation, the physical comfort of the table, the security of her environment, and her trust in those caring for her.

The unnatural position of the patient's legs in stirrups in addition to decreased muscle power and skeletal changes may make it difficult for the elderly patient to sit up after the examination without assistance. Unassisted, she will attempt to roll on her side for necessary leverage with her elbow in order to rise to a sitting position. The narrowness of the table makes this a dangerous attempt.

Excitement, embarrassment, or anxiety desensitizes a patient to verbal and nonverbal cues. She may hear part or no part of the initial instructions to prepare for or terminate the examination. Rather than make a mistake, she may then helplessly sit down and hope the nurse will enter and save her embarrassment. Instructions to patients are most likely to be heard and understood if given slowly, distinctly enunciated in sufficient volume, and repeated without irritation or censure.

GYNECOLOGIC PROBLEMS OF THE OLDER PATIENT

Some of the most commonly seen gynecologic problems of the older patient are due to decreased muscle tone, tissue changes, and obstetric trauma, with prolapse of the uterus, cystocele, and rectocele. Malignant lesions are also found in the older woman.

Relaxation lesions. The patient with relaxation lesions has the feeling of something falling, a dragging sensation, and pressure. Associated with these feelings are those of apprehension and embarrassment, not knowing what is happening to her and yet also knowing that there is a very abnormal protrusion. She may have dribbling of urine, urgency and frequency, nocturia, and stress incontinence, all of which accentuate her apprehensions. She may feel so insecure that she begins to wear a sanitary napkin to prevent soiling her clothing. "I feel embarrassed to buy them in the store. I never thought I'd ever wear those things again." Associated with this may be a persistent urine smell.

Herbs were used as remedial treatment of uterine prolapse in the fifth and sixth century to try to reduce the size of the prolapse and to heal the ulcerations that were commonly present. All else failing, amputation of the extended part was performed. Pessaries have been in use since the days of Hippocrates, who wrote of those made of bone.

Proper obstetric care may decrease the incidence of these lesions. Prophylactic measures include good prenatal care, which leads to fewer complications during labor and delivery, prevention of prolonged labor and the proper timing and use of obstetric forceps and episiotomy, and immediate and late postpartum care. In spite of excellent obstetric care, relaxation lesions may occur, since the most important factors are the patient's own tissue integrity, elasticity, and nutrition.

Cystocele. Cystocele is a protrusion of the bladder, with marked thinning or an actual defect in the pubocervical fascia. Symptoms, which depend on the size and any coexisting lesion, are usually bearing-down discomfort, the sensation of a mass protruding from the vagina or of the organs falling out, and urinary disability such as stress incontinence. These symptoms are enhanced during activity such as walking, standing, or other forms of physical exercise. Upon physical examination a bulging of the anterior vaginal wall and usually a coexisting urethrocele (bulging of the urethra) and uterine prolapse are found. The patient is examined in lithotomy position and also in standing position to demonstrate the presence of cystocele, uterine prolapse, rectocele, and possible enterocele (protrusion of the bowel into the vagina).

Treatment depends on the size of lesions and severity of symptoms as well as the presence of coexisting lesions. Small lesions that are asymptomatic usually require no treatment. If there are distressing symptoms and coexisting lesions such as prolapse, enterocele, rectocele, and urethrocele, then surgical repair is usually indicated. Large lesions, either symptomatic or asymptomatic, should be repaired unless there is a medical contraindication or a coexisting carcinoma of the genital tract. Treatment consists of dissection of the bladder and the anterior vaginal walls and repair of the fascial defect. This is often accompanied by vaginal hysterectomy.

Urethrocele. Urethrocele, a urethral protrusion into the vagina, is the result of injury of the urogenital diaphragm and pubocervical fascia, with detachment of the vesicle neck and urethra from their normal position beneath the pubic bone. This interferes with function, and the usual symptom is urinary stress incontinence (loss of urine with coughing or sneezing). The defect is seen as a small bulging of the urethra; it is differentiated from a urethral diverticulum or cyst. Treatment is surgical and is based on fixation of the vesicle neck in its normal position in support of the urethra. As a primary procedure, vaginal repair is performed; if this is unsuccessful, an abdominal procedure, the Marshall-Marchetti-Krantz procedure, is indicated. Any coexisting relaxation lesion should be repaired at the same time.

Uterine prolapse. Uterine prolapse is a variable degree of descent of the uterus, with overstretching of the uterine supports. The symptoms are a bearing-down sensation and protrusion of the cervix or the entire uterus through the vagina. It is usually associated with cystocele and rectocele and the symptoms thereof. (Fig. 11.) Treatment in the older patient is vaginal hysterectomy and repair. In the younger patient who desires more children, operation is usually deferred until the family is complete. If symptoms are severe, a Manchester type of operation (repair of the cystocele and vaginal support of the uterus) may be done in younger patients.

Rectocele. Rectocele is a posterior wall lesion, with protrusion of the rectum into the vagina. This is usually asymptomatic. Occasionally the patient notes a bulging mass or an inability to evacuate the rectum without splinting the vagina. Physical examination reveals a forward, outward bulging of the posterior vaginal wall. This must be differentiated from an enterocele. Treatment is frequently not required. If there are coexisting lesions of prolapse and cystocele that demand treatment, the rectocele is repaired at the same time.

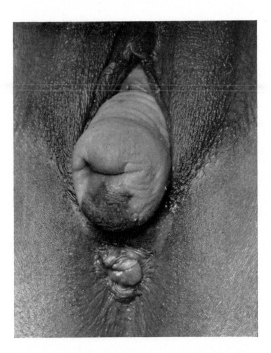

Fig. 11. Procidentia, showing protrusion of the uterus and bladder through the vagina.

Enterocele. Enterocele is a hernia between the rectum, the uterosacral ligaments, and the posterior surface of the uterus. It is a true hernia, having a peritoneal sac that may contain loops of small intestine or omentum. Usually there is accompanying uterine prolapse, cystocele, and rectocele and these lesions should all be repaired at the same time.

Until symptoms become severe, the older patient may not seek help for relaxation lesions. She may feel she is too old for surgery or that she should not bother with this examination and treatment at her age.

Postmenopausal bleeding. Postmenopausal bleeding is resumption of bleeding one or more years after the last normal menstrual period. These patients must all be evaluated. A very high percentage (25 to 60%) may have uterine cancer. (Even bleeding following hormone therapy is suspicious.) This figure is being lowered as more patients with postmenopausal bleeding are being hospitalized and diagnostic procedures are performed. Of patients admitted to Passavant Memorial Hospital in Chicago for postmenopausal bleeding, 27.5% had carcinoma, 34.1% had benign lesions, and 38.4% had no demonstrable lesions.

Neither the quantity, the character, nor the duration of bleeding can distinguish benign from malignant lesions. All patients with postmenopausal bleeding should have a cytosmear, diagnostic curettage, and cervical biopsy. Usually this is adequate treatment. If bleeding continues or recurs following the curettement, a second curettage should be done. If no lesion is found at this time, a hysterectomy is indicated. The diagnostic curettage is not infallible, with an approximate 6% error in the diagnosis of malignancy. If there are coexisting relaxation lesions and if no malignancy is discovered, hysterectomy may be done by choice. When definitive treatment is not done and bleeding recurs, the patient must be reevaluated and definitively treated.

Leukoplakia and kraurosis of the vulva. Tissue changes in the elderly patient predispose her to vulvar lesions such as leukoplakia, kraurosis, and carcinoma. The symptoms are similar, with itching, dryness of the skin, and dyspareunia. Fissuring or ulceration occurs, with secondary infection usually due to scratching. In patients with carcinoma of the vulva 60% have an associated leukoplakia and 40% have associated kraurosis. The converse of this is not known—that is, how many patients with leukoplakic vulvitis develop carcinoma. Although it is a very small percentage, there is definite danger.

Leukoplakia, which means "white plaque," may be either a white lesion of the mucous membrane of the vulva or it may be red, gray, or blue. It may be present either alone or in conjunction with kraurosis and/or carcinoma. Since there may be a variety of colors, actual diagnosis of leukoplakia must be made by microscopic examination of tissue that is obtained by biopsy.

Kraurosis is also a white lesion that often involves the labia and the tissues about the clitoris. The skin is usually thin and parchmentlike in appearance, with frequent fissuring and ulceration. Although this is an atrophic lesion, carcinoma may develop. Biopsy and microscopic examination are necessary to differentiate this from other lesions of the vulva such as lichen sclerosis et atrophicus and senile atrophy.

Many forms of therapy have been used, such as wet dressings, hormones, oils, or vitamins, but with little success. For both leukoplakia and kraurosis, vulvectomy is the procedure of choice, and if the symptoms are severe, it is recommended.

It should be pointed out that simple vulvectomy, which removes the skin of the vulva, labia majora and minora, and clitoris, does not destroy vaginal function and often does not interfere with normal sex life.

Carcinoma of the vulva. Carcinoma of the vulva is a relatively rare malignancy occurring most frequently in the older age group. It is usually a squamous cell carcinoma arising from the skin or mucous membrane of the vulva, from a pre-existing leukoplakia or kraurosis, from the urethra, or from the Bartholin gland or sweat gland or a melanocarcinoma arising in a nevus (Fig. 12). Intraepithelial carcinoma (carcinoma in situ) also occurs on the vulva. While this stage is curable, it has been known to progress to invasive carcinoma.

Early symptoms of carcinoma of the vulva may be pruritus followed by sore-

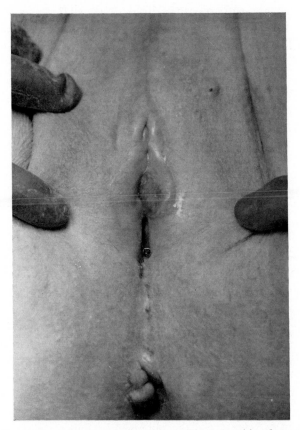

Fig. 12. Squamous cell carcinoma of the vulva. Other atrophic changes in the external genitalia may also be seen in this older woman.

ness, bloody discharge, and a mass. Early spread to the regional lymph nodes is common, particularly the inguinal and iliac nodes. Treatment is radical vulvectomy (wider and deeper resection than simple vulvectomy) and bilateral removal of the deep and superficial lymph nodes. Because this disease usually occurs in post-climacteric women who are frequently poor operative risks, the operation is often done in stages rather than all at once. X-ray therapy is of little value.

The patient following vulvectomy. Because of the extent of the operation, the patient's age, and coexisting medical problems, these patients need help. The convalescence is frequently prolonged in the hospital because of drainage from the wound site. It is often difficult to close the entire incision and the danger of repeated urethral catheterization is ever present. The patient's convalescent course often is discouraging to her.

Movement and ambulation may be difficult for the patient who has had a vulvectomy. She may require frequent pain relief. Vulvar pain involves cutaneous rather than somatic pathways and the patient describes her pain as burning and stinging. It is often considered desirable to administer analgesics prior to ambulation, since sitting and moving into a sitting position are very painful. Time and patience are nursing essentials as the patient slowly shifts her weight from side to side and inches close to the edge of the bed to sit up or as she slowly maneuvers back into bed. This patient often tends to lie in one position, fearful to move and cause more pain. The most considerate care given her is extended *very early,* showing her the ease of turning by shifting weight from one hip to the other and how to move up and down in bed *without* reaching overhead and grasping the head of the bed.

Lack of privacy is a constant fear for this patient. Because she receives perineal care frequently to make her more comfortable and to reduce the odor usually present, the patient is wary of both doors and screens, even though closed, knowing well that most people in the hospital open the door and screen first and announce themselves later. An even greater fear exists when she is left alone with a perineal lamp in position. Though she feels its benefits of pain relief and comfort in the operated site, her fear of exposure may force her to refuse the lamp. If some unexpected visitor should arrive, she would be in a most awkward and embarrassing situation. Many patients are unwilling to chance it. They can be reassured by careful attention to draping, screening, and the protection of a sign on the door.

Of all gynecologic procedures performed on the elderly person, vulvectomy, by its visible reinforcement, is the most mutilating. The woman who has had a hysterectomy may *think* of herself as different, as a "shell of a woman," but the patient with a vulvectomy can both see and feel that she is different. Nurses also react to this gynecologic amputation. They feel that the patients are difficult to care for and complain that the smell bothers them. The patients too are sensitively aware of an odor and are especially apprehensive when family and visitors are present. They also apologize to the nurse for the presence of the odor.

Two vulvectomy patients, good preoperative hospital friends, seemed to be at swords' points most of the time during their convalescent period. They vied with one another for attention and carried on a running war of insults and thinly veiled humor. After they were moved to separate rooms, one patient confided her fear that the personnel soon would have bypassed her room because the smell was too unpleasant. She felt she could in some measure control herself but could not tolerate the duplicated problem in another. The other patient similarly expressed her worry of their compounded problem. Separated, both were more relaxed and able to enjoy their families. Both were particularly prepared and anxious for company when they were given perineal care immediately before visitors were expected.

FACTORS INFLUENCING HOSPITALIZATION AND POSTOPERATIVE CARE OF THE ELDERLY GYNECOLOGIC PATIENT

Even though a woman is long past the childbearing years, she may still have strong feelings about the loss of her uterus by surgical means and still equate the uterus with femininity. The elderly patient may be no more apprehensive than any other patient, or she may have more resources than a young patient who has not the time or the will to face a nebulous future. The elderly patient may feel she is physically vulnerable when she hears, "Anyone who can do a full day's work can tolerate an anesthetic," or "As long as your heart's OK, you have nothing to fear." A student remembered:

I think the thing that frightened her most was the thought of the anesthetic. She was once told that if she had any trouble with her heart she should never have gas. I told her before she went down that she would get an anesthetic in the arm. "Is it bad for my heart?" and I said, "No." She said she realized they improved a lot of things in medicine, but she didn't think they had improved anesthetics since the twenties when she had her last operation.

The ability of the aged person to tolerate any procedure is dependent on the efficiency of the vital organs—brain, heart, lungs, liver, and kidney—and the adrenocortical response to stress. The heart, brain, and kidneys are the most vulnerable to degenerative changes. Prior to operation an evaluation of vital organs and stress reserves is important to determine medical, anesthesia, and postoperative care. In the presence of degenerative changes the responses to trauma may be overwhelmed by edema, hypoproteinemia, or congestive heart failure.

The postoperative care of the aging individual necessitates nursing vigilance and knowledge based on the physiologic and psychologic changes present before surgery, the trauma of the surgery experience, and these effects on the particular older individual involved. Safe and effective nursing judgments are more apt to be made with possession of such knowledge. Specific problems of the aged gynecologic patient who has had an operation are considered here. Problems common to many age groups are to be found in Chapters 3 and 4.

Stress reserves vs. stressors. Stress reserves are low in the aging person. To all changes in homeostasis, response and adaptive reactions tend to be slow and less vigorous, and thus responses to stress of illness and injury are subtle, insidious, and easily obscured and overlooked. The usually observed and expected signs and symptoms or complications may be entirely lacking, so modified that their importance is difficult to ascertain, or so minimal that safe evaluation is sometimes improbable. A two-day period of malaise may explode into a fulminating cystitis or into terminal pneumonia. Vague discomfort may herald acute urinary retention, paralytic ileus, or wound disruption. A slower, narrower margin of homeostatic regulation against disease processes and environmental demands means that the aging person is more vulnerable and more quickly overwhelmed by dehydration, water intoxication, circulatory overloading, starvation, extremes of temperature, and pain.

Dehydration, water intoxication, or overloading. Loss of water because of emesis, diarrheal stools, and gastric suction dehydrates the aging individual rapidly. She not only does not immediately adapt to water-losing situations but she is also not able to compensate easily for the losses from her own tissues when aging muscle, cutaneous fat, and intra- and extracellular water are diminished. Replacement of water is usually essential for the older patient.

Overloading with too many fluids or too rapidly administered fluids demands immediate cardiac measures and renal regulation. This adaptation may not be possible in the elderly patient in the presence of decreased cardiac and renal tubular efficiency. This means that the fluids given an aging individual may have to be regulated and controlled by blood pressure, pulse determinations, and other observations of the patient to prevent pulmonary edema.

Starvation. The reserves of protein and fat are reduced in the aged person, with diminished possibility of self-restoring food stores when these are imperative for energy and wound restoration. When the gastrointestinal tract is again mobile, small and frequent meals should be encouraged. These should be high in protein and vitamin C for wound healing and the restoration of body reserves. Some older patients have diminished food tastes, especially salty and sour. Since sweet taste remains, their choice of food may reflect a preference for carbohydrates. The aging patient may have further difficulties of faulty dentition and deglutition and may refuse meat in her diet. Usually women patients wear their dentures if they have them. More frequently, patients neglect to wear partial plates or bridges that do not show but that are essential for adequate mastication of food and ease of swallowing.

A vacillating appetite and early fatigue may turn a lunch period into certain defeat as the patient views large quantities of food and a large piece of meat, as yet uncut. Preparation of food for the early postoperative aging patient frees fleeting energy for the enjoyment of food. The success of the Meals-on-Wheels program in the homes of elderly persons has successfully demonstrated the beneficial influence of "company" on the appetite of the solitary individual. Its message might be kept in mind for the many convalescent patients of all ages who sit alone in their private rooms for three meals a day. Occasionally at least, these patients may welcome the opportunity to eat with some of the other patients they meet. The social aspects of eating are important to patients. It would be interesting to contemplate the many other positive benefits patients could have on one another.

Extremes of temperature. As with the very young, the aging patient has decreased defenses against temperature extremes. The patient's decreased apocrine secretion and the decreased response to stress result in decreased perspiration and decreased regulatory responses to temperature changes in the external environment or to the internal environment of fever. Body temperature may rise rapidly and unabated, and the aged person may become rapidly overheated. Hospital rooms with poor air circulation provide further insult to the individual with increased heat retention. Environmental control for the elderly patient in summer is important.

They also have decreased heat production in response to cold. In a study conducted in 1960 of persons aged 60 to 80 years it is reported that only one out of every ten elderly well individuals responded with any increase in production of body heat and metabolism when exposed to a temperature of 48° F. All failed to start shivering after 40 to 45 minutes' exposure, while younger subjects responded with three to four times metabolic heat production.*

Such inabilities to cope with temperature changes are important factors to consider for medical intervention with ice and alcohol sponges and the applications of external heat. The vulnerability of these individuals to these treatments without usual defenses of regulation is seldom acknowledged.

Pain. Pain is not always readily identified by the patient, and some studies indicate a pain decrement in the aging patient. Other studies do not seem to substantiate this finding. Whether the older patient has a changed intake component or whether there is a difference in the pain processing component, that is, if the patient does not complain of her pain as readily (Chapter 2), pain is expensive on energy and metabolic adjustments. Renal and cardiac activity is influenced by the prolonged presence of pain. Thus recognition and evaluation of pain and provision for its relief with safe and effective analgesics are conservation as well as humanitarian measures. Confusion, apathy, or other manifestations of *oversedation* are also detrimental to the convalescence of the patient and are just as costly to her welfare as the pain. The recurring evaluations and wise judgments of the nurse are essential.

Energy demands vs. fatigue. The aging patient may have difficulty getting out of bed. Weakness, diminished muscle tone, and pain may impede her independent movement and she may require assistance longer than other patients. Usually this may involve assisting her to a sitting position. After that she can take care of herself. She usually will find it easier to roll to the side and then get to a sitting position with her legs over the side of the bed.

Response to the surgical stresses may be manifest as perspiration, fluctuating blood pressure, and dizziness when the patient is ambulated for the first time. There is wide variance in the physiologic functioning of the cardiovascular system

---

*United States Department of Health, Education, and Welfare: Vital statistics of the United States, Washington, D. C., 1960, U.S. Government Printing Office.

in different individuals. This being so, helping the patient out of bed at least during the first few postoperative days requires close nursing observation.

Even before helping the patient out of bed, the nurse has made many objective and subjective observations. She has a basal evaluation of the patient's blood pressure. She has evaluated the quality and regularity of the pulse at rest and after the activities of turning and experiences of pain. She has evaluated her color and the presence of perspiration at rest and after exertion. She has also evaluated the patient's readiness or reticence to relate the presence of pain, her accuracy of description, or her poverty of expression regarding pain and other physical discomforts. The fact that a patient gets out of bed at all the first few days postoperation speaks for her compliance to nursing directives. This means that a patient depends on and trusts nursing judgment to control the situation and to regulate its safety for her. The patient who has had previous pain and shortness of breath may assume the nurse will remember it and that it is all right or expected. After all, she had these same feelings at rest when the nurse checked her blood pressure and pulse, and she still told her to get out of bed.

In addition to increased alertness for untoward signs of intolerance to ambulation in the elderly person, the patient needs to be rescued from the fatigue of the maneuver. During the first few postoperative days she becomes easily tired and discouraged. Shorter and more frequent periods of ambulation are indicated rather than one long one that creates dread for the next venture. It is far wiser to assist her back to bed while she still feels strong enough to stay up longer and may even feel she is stronger than she thought possible. For a weak aged patient it is doubtful if forceful "removal" from bed just to say she has been up is of any benefit in either providing circulatory changes or minimizing a reducing muscle mass. Inactivity in a chair may be more restricting than a bed and may only *increase* pelvic stasis and possible phlebitis. For such a patient effective deep breathing, moving about in bed, and passive and active exercising in bed may be far more important for improvement in circulatory changes and improved muscle tone.

Environmental stresses. Perhaps more than any other patient the newly admitted aging patient requires frequent contact with understanding hospital personnel. Unnoticed and unattended, apprehension and depression in the elderly patient may result in the frequent *confusion* of the newly admitted patient or the new postoperative patient. It has been noted that patients who enter the hospital from an isolated type of living are more prone to acute confusion. Diminishing sensory perception in addition to diminishing important human contacts results in symptoms of sensory deprivation. These take the form of sensory distortions and then apprehension because of the distortions, confusion because of the inability to interpret the distorted sensory stimuli to the present situation, and finally mounting excitement because of the whole stressful event. Unfocused thought and disconnected bits of memory aroused by sensory stimuli may further frighten the patient and emphasize that she is not in control.

The nurse in contact with the patient for an eight-hour period and the nursing staff in general, having the opportunity of continuous contact with the patient for 24 hours, can function as vital interpretors to a patient in a strange environment. They can act as an amplifier to the patient whose sensory percepts are recording hazy pictures, dulled sounds, or inaccurate awareness of position. For example:

Mrs. Smith was frequently confused for two days after her abdominal hysterectomy. She forgot where she was, was not aware that the surgery was over, did not recognize known nurses, and was visibly excited and agitated with her incision, its dressing, the Foley catheter, and genitourinary tubing. She rolled back and forth against the side rails, moaning continuously. Only in retrospect did the nurses and personnel recall the preoperative instances when this older patient had misplaced her personal belongings, had become excited, had used someone else's blanket or robe, and occasionally had lost her way to her room. Hospital personnel had joked with her and considered her "a cute little thing." Her problems had been overlooked or whitewashed. The patient as a person had been devalued.

Factors that singly or in combination cause confusional states in *any* individual are shown in Fig. 13. Because of coexisting changes of age the elderly patient is more vulnerable to increased physiologic disabilities or any increased stress situation.

Confusion in the elderly person may be observed as a diurnal variation. Confusion in the evening hours is often due to changes in the auditory, visual, and proprioceptive faculties secondary to fatigue. Often there is an alteration in her ability for dark adaption and to see at various degrees of illumination. This necessitates better reading lights and *more* light for eating and night lights than seem necessary for younger patients. At night the aging person may see only shadowy forms that make any special interpretation of room size or furniture forms difficult.

Often there is also a diminution of hearing. This may not involve hearing conversation or the comprehension of language. It may, however, involve all background noises, noises such as doors opening and closing, footsteps approaching, and any other such sound that constantly and sometimes unconsciously keeps an individual safely aware of her surroundings and herself in it. The patient with this hearing deficiency may often be unaware of the exact loss. The patient's ability to orient herself within her surroundings is severely reduced when a diminished level of background noises is coupled with indistinguishable night shadows and diminished tactile and proprioceptive abilities. The patient may be fearful of a strange formless shadow and may not accurately feel the edge of the table or the middle of the footstool as she tries to leave her bed in the dark. She may be enveloped in hushed silence. Her coordination may not be good enough to prevent falling. Fear and confusion often result.

This implies that communication with the patient at night should be well chosen in order to orient and reassure her. It also indicates that whispering will be unheard or misinterpreted and will sooner or later necessitate a volume that *can* be heard. Nursing personnel should be visible to this patient without the visual distortions made by a flashlight. Other nursing controls for the older patient include

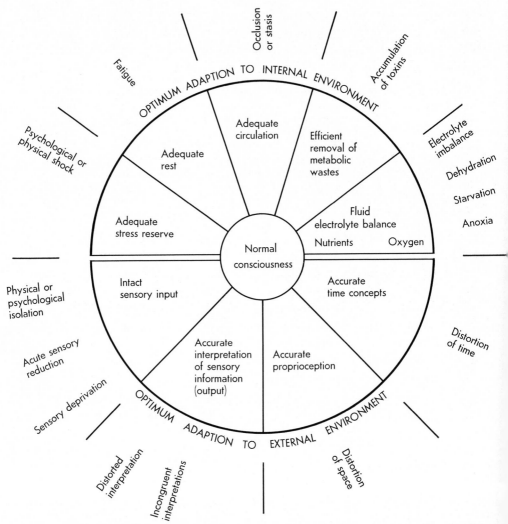

Fig. 13. Factors involved in confusional states. The factors that must be present in all individuals (or a satisfactory adaptation) if they are to be in a state of equilibrium with their internal and external environment are shown in the center wheel. The absence or distortion of any of these factors is indicated peripheral to the wheel. Inadequate compensation or inappropriate adaptations by the patient when any vital factors are distorted will result in confusion and disorientation. The nurse is able to control and regulate many of these factors for the patient. She is able to observe signs of early distortion and augment the patient's abilities to compensate.

maintenance of a stable environment so that the bed, table, and other furniture are always in the same place and that obstacles such as intravenous stands are removed. It is advisable that this patient be given a room prior to operation that she can remain in for the duration of the hospitalization to maintain familiar points of reference, that is, window placement, door, etc. The presence of the family and their bridge with the home are most important to maintain the patient's freedom

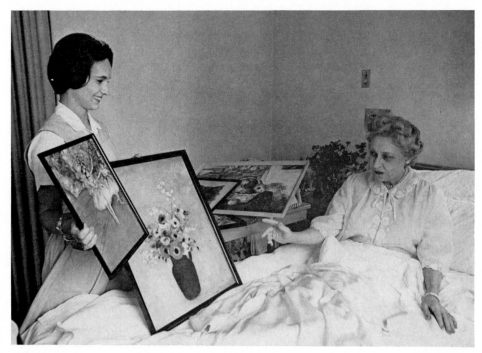

Fig. 14. Pictures help to bring "home" to the hospital. The belief that the patient's environment can affect her therapy prompts many forms of action. Here a volunteer offers a patient a wide selection of pictures from her "art cart." (Courtesy Passavant Memorial Hospital, Chicago, Ill.)

from confusion. A further bridge with the home is afforded when the patient is able to see a few of her own possessions on her bedside table or overbed stand. Colorful, light rooms can reduce the effects of the physical stresses of her hospitalization and can minimize depression. Some hospitals provide art reproductions that may be hung in the hospital room. These are selected by the patient and changed as frequently as she wishes to make a new selection. (Fig. 14.)

Sleeping medications may be undesirable for the aged patient since they tend to accumulate in tissues and result in oversedation or restlessness. Evening confusion, fears, and restlessness may well be laid to the use of barbiturates in aging patients. Chloral hydrate, an old medication, is being reevaluated and seems to be an excellent evening sedation for the elderly.

The effects of physical restraints in creating and increasing a confusion state are well known. Studies of sensory deprivation substantiate these clinical observations.

Interpersonal stresses. Only in circumstances of common disaster, war, flood, tornado, hurricane, and *hospitalization* are individuals placed in a situation where they are required to sleep, eat, bathe, and attend toilet necessities in constant proximity to total strangers.

Since hospital personnel tend to be intolerant to evidences of strife or disagreement of these "strangers" forced to live together, patients discipline one another to minimize censure and try to become "good" patients. In one hospital study* new patients admitted to a clinical unit were found to learn quickly those things that displeased nurses, dietitians, ward attendants, and other patients. Among these were any disturbances in the ward, unnecessary noise, criticism of the ward or staff, rebellion against routine, overcomplaining, or overconcern. It has been identified that patients frequently test out the hospital staff in an attempt to determine who they are and what can be expected of them. Another study has reported that "a frequent and often unnamed [patient] fear was that an 'angered' staff *would retaliate by withdrawing aid when the patient needed it most.*"† (Italics ours.)

It is no wonder that the older patient often has a difficult orientation to the hospital situation. Testing behavior of the older patient is frequent and may be identified in the form of demanding, excessive talking, or often a reluctance to release a new-found audience. The older patient cannot always fit the definition of a "good" patient if by "good" is meant the patient should be able to conform to routine without undue complaint. To do so implies the presence of a certain amount of passive and permissive behavior. To an aging individual the harrowing effects of illness arouse fears, worries, and self-concern. Complaining is a desired and expressive sequela. Flexible adjustments to completely new situations are not common for elderly persons, who in turn see little justification for hospital rigidities and nursing inflexibilities. Most important, passivity in elderly persons in a stressful situation is equated with hopelessness. The active demanding older patient, with signs of fight and active desires to participate in her own convalescence, are to be desired. These attributes, however, often do not fit the mold of the "model" patient, more often called the "cooperative" patient.

Who do we consider the cooperative patient? Student nurses make the following comments:

> Sometimes if a patient just says 'thank you' for some of the little things you do that other patients don't notice, you think this patient is cooperative. Maybe she actually isn't, but it's appreciation.

> I think nurses term a 'cooperative' patient as one to whom they can say, 'OK, stand now, I want to do this; sit down now, I want to do this.' Unfortunately, we consider her cooperative if she does what we want her to do, regardless of whether it's what she herself wants to do or what she should be doing.

> If she doesn't bother us we think she is cooperative.

> A cooperative patient is one who will do what should be done when you explain it to her. Then she can do what she really wants to do.

---

*Schottstaedt, William W., Pinsky, Ruth H., Mackler, David, and Wolf, Stewart: Sociologic, psychologic and metabolic observations on patients in the community of a metabolic ward, American Journal of Medicine **25**:248-257, 1958.

†Visotsky, Harold M., Hamburg, David A., Goss, Mary E., and Lebovits, Binyamin Z.: Coping behavior under extreme stress, Archives of General Psychiatry **5**:431-432, 1961.

If someone demands something she's able to do for herself, I think she's uncooperative. If a person is ill and requires a lot of time and demands your attention, I don't
think that person is uncooperative.

These nurses' opinions of the cooperative patient are substantiated by Visotsky's observations. "There is a range of behavior typical for sick patients, and
therapeutic personnel come to expect that all patients will fall within this range.
Those who deviate from it are likely to be viewed with suspicion or even animos-
ity."* The staff appreciates a patient who does not bother them. They often consider a patient content when she is compliant. The staff likes friendliness in a patient, an appreciation of staff efforts, patience, understanding of staff problems,
and a sense of humor.* *"In general, staff members expect and need a high level
of respect from patients."**

Older patients are therefore exposed not only to illness and injury stresses and
to the environmental demands of changing situations but also to continuing strains
of maintaining and enhancing important interpersonal relationships of those upon
whom they must depend.

To value any patient is to respect her as a human being. She is included in
those events and conversation that involve her present and future life. Actions
toward her involve feelings of goodwill; she is not manipulated for the secondary
gains or satisfactions of nursing personnel under the guise of "It's for her own
good."

The relationship of interdependence with the older patient, her family, and the
helping professions offers the optimum therapeutic environment in which *all* individuals are most able to realize their potential abilities, strengths, and powers
of extended giving to others. This implies an empathic relationship with a patient
founded in respect and goodwill which seeks mutual understanding through conscious identification. It is imagining what the patient is like and comparing something about her with something similar and different in yourself or someone previously known. This leads to *some* understanding and knowledge of the other person. Probably the greatest misunderstanding of the empathic process is its essential
of *mutuality*. Nurses utilize many means to learn about patients: rogerian interviewing techniques, process recordings, case studies, and conferences. However,
the mutual knowing of patient *and* nurse is often absent. In other words, the knowing is all one-sided: all toward knowing only the patient. Its purpose is to get information and to understand the patient *so that* nursing care can be planned. Unless this purpose is motivated by feelings of goodwill to the particular patient and
unless it lacks the desire to control the patient for the secondary gains of the nurse
or so she can carry out her nursing plan more completely, the process is not really
empathy. The same process may be practiced by a zealous enemy on his victim
who also seeks "to know" so that he may control and devise strategy.† Empathy is

---

*Visotsky, Harold M., Hamburg, David A., Goss, Mary E., and Lebovits, Binyamin Z.:
Coping behavior under extreme stress, Archives of General Psychiatry, **5:**432, 1961.

†Stewart, David A.: Preface to empathy. New York, 1956, Philosophical Library Inc.

not the means toward an end. It is the ongoing process that includes *all* individuals in the relationship. It is awareness of self in the relationship. It is trust and concern for another as a respected individual of worth. Such relationships are therapeutic for all ages.

RECOMMENDED READINGS FOR STUDENTS

Bettelheim, Bruno: The problem of generations. In Erikson, Erik, editor: Youth: change and challenge, New York, 1963, Basic Books, Inc., Publishers, pp. 64-92.

Kogan, Nathan, and Shelton, Florence C.: Beliefs about "old people": A comparative study of older and younger samples, Journal of Genetic Psychology **100:**93-111, 1962.

Neisser, Marianne: The two must face a third, Social Casework **39**(1)27-29, 1958. (Although written for the student social worker, this article is pertinent for the student nurse and her instructor when "nurse" is substituted for "worker" and "patient" is substituted for "client.")

Orlando, Ida Jean: The dynamic nurse-patient relationship, New York, 1961, G. P. Putnam's Sons.

Peplau, Hildegard E.: Loneliness, American Journal of Nursing **55:**1477-1481, 1955.

Phillips, Elisabeth Cogswell: Meals a la car, Nursing Outlook **8**(2):76-78, 1960.

Ruesch, Jurgen, and Kees, Weldon: Non-verbal communication: Notes on the visual perception of human relations, Berkeley, 1964, University of California Press.

RECOMMENDED READINGS FOR INSTRUCTORS AND THE EXCEPTIONAL STUDENT

Brewer, John I.: Textbook of gynecology, Baltimore, 1961, The Williams & Wilkins Co.

Brewer, John I., and Miller, W. H.: Postmenopausal uterine bleeding, American Journal of Obstetrics and Gynecology **67:**988-1013, 1954.

Jackman, Norman, Schottstaedt, William, McPhail, S. Clark., and Wolf, Stewart: Interaction, emotion and physiologic change, Journal of Health and Human Behavior **4:**83-87, 1963.

Moore, Francis D.: Metabolic care of the surgical patient, Philadelphia, 1959, W. B. Saunders Co., pp. 71-72, 840, 845.

Schwartz, William: Ambivalent mother surrogate, Psychosomatics **3:**484-486, 1962.

Stewart, David A.: Preface to empathy, New York, 1956, Philosophical Library, Inc.

Sturgis, Somers H., et al.: The gynecologic patient, a psycho-endocrine study, New York, 1962, Grune & Stratton, Inc.

Titchener, James, et al.: Psychological reactions of the aged in surgery, A. M. A. Archives of Neuro-Psychiatry **79:**63-73, 1958.

Chapter 8

The patient with gynecologic malignancy

The establishment of an early diagnosis of malignancy leads to early treatment and a high cure rate. This chapter on the malignancies of the female genitalia is begun with this optimistic viewpoint since a major problem in effective treatment is delay. While technical problems of surgical excision, radiation, and chemotherapy still exist, the prognosis is largely determined by the extent of the disease as well as the biologic nature of the disease when it is first encountered. Relatively simple diagnostic procedures may be used because of the easy accessibility of the female genitalia.

Cancers of the vulva, vagina, and cervix are easily inspected and palpated. Diagnostic Papanicolaou smears and biopsies are readily taken. Cancer of the endometrium, though slightly less accessible, may be found by biopsy, by endometrial and Papanicolaou smear, by instruments, and by curettage. Systematic periodic examinations aid in the early discovery of ovarian tumors, for these remain symptomless until late in the disease. Early invasive carcinoma of the cervix should be 85 to 95% curable if found when less than 1 cm. in diameter; if it is found in its preinvasive phase, it is nearly 100% curable. An early diagnosis of cancer of the endometrium may result in equally good cure rates.

Vaginal bleeding is the principal symptom of uterine cancer that causes a patient to seek medical attention. Unfortunately, bleeding from a malignancy has no distinguishing characteristics from nonmalignant sources of bleeding. Any abnormal bleeding must be investigated so that a malignancy will not be neglected. As discussed in Chapter 6, any uterine bleeding between menstrual periods or postcoital bleeding indicates the possible presence of carcinoma of the uterus. The latter suggests carcinoma of the cervix. Postmenopausal bleeding may mean a uterine malignancy, either endometrial or cervical. Pain occurs very late and is often a symptom of some complication or extension of the disease.

PATIENT DELAY

A recent study* has indicated that, of the seven warning symptoms emphasized by the American Cancer Society, the symptom of unusual bleeding or discharge was ignored by the patient for the longest time before seeking medical advice. Forty-two percent of the population tested waited longer than three months before seeking help. Another study† concluded that patients seek medical advice for ambiguous symptoms, for those present a long time, and for illness that interferes with their activity. If these observations also pertain to the gynecologic patient, it is apparent that she must be educated to the recognition and interpretation of her symptoms when they arise. That is, she must be educated to realize the importance of seeking medical advice, even if the symptoms occur only once or infrequently. She must have faith in her doctor's ability to help her and assurance of his patience and approval of her, even if her "symptoms" fail to indicate anything abnormal and her fears prove unfounded. Patients today are made acutely aware of the "busy" doctor and therefore hesitate to make appointments or to sit in busy waiting rooms unless they are sure something is wrong.

The gynecologic patient may wait for several months until she can discern and report a pattern of abnormal bleeding, discharge, abdominal enlargement, or other recurrent symptoms. Greater surety of maintaining health by providing early treatment for disease can be accomplished through periodic gynecologic examinations of women of all ages. This should be a semiannual examination. Such convictions sincerely held by the nurse herself can be incorporated into her health teaching to the patient, neighbor, or friend. Because of her influence a future periodic examination may avert the insidious progression of a malignancy.

Carcinoma of cervix

The most frequent malignancy of the female genital tract is carcinoma of the cervix. It is exceeded in frequency only by carcinoma of the breast. Approximately 2% or more of women will have carcinoma of the cervix before the age of 80 years. While carcinoma of the cervix is generally reported to be three to six times more common than endometrial carcinoma, at Passavant Memorial Hospital in Chicago the ratio is 1.5 cervical to 1 endometrial malignancy. It occurs more frequently in women who marry early and who have children early in life. It is also more frequent in non-Jewish women. It occurs less frequently in the nulliparous woman. It is much less common in those who live a celibate type of life.

---

*Apple, Dorrian: How laymen define illness, Journal of Health and Human Behavior **1:** 219-225, 1960.

†Kutner, Bernard, and Gordon, Gerald: Seeking cure for cancer, Journal of Health and Human Behavior **2:**171-178, 1961.

Carcinoma of the cervix may occur at any age, although it is predominantly seen between the ages of 40 and 50 years.

Because the cervix is readily accessible to visual, digital, and cytologic examinations, cancer of the cervix theoretically might cease to be a major health problem if every woman had a routine gynecologic examination regularly and if she notified her doctor at any sign of abnormal bleeding or leukorrhea.

It is impossible either visually or by palpation to diagnose preinvasive or minimal invasive carcinoma of the cervix, since both are present before any signs and symptoms are produced. Therefore, a cytologic smear (Papanicolaou) should be obtained on each patient. These smears have been shown to be 95% accurate in carcinoma of the cervix and approximately 75% accurate in carcinoma of the endometrium. A positive or abnormal smear indicates only that abnormal cells have been seen on the slide and that there is a possibility that carcinoma exists. It cannot indicate whether this carcinoma is invasive or preinvasive. Therefore, an abnormal smear indicates only that further diagnostic procedures must be done. These include biopsy of the cervix, a possible conization of the cervix, and curettage of the endocervical and endometrial canals.

Carcinoma in situ. When malignant cellular changes are limited to the epithelial layer and when there is no invasion below this layer into the stroma of the tissue, the lesion is called carcinoma in situ. Other names applied to this lesion are intraepithelial carcinoma, preinvasive carcinoma, noninvasive carcinoma, surface carcinoma, Bowen's disease, preclinical carcinoma, subclinical carcinoma, and stage 0 carcinoma of the cervix. The name signifies that the lesion is the early phase of tissue changes from normal to abnormal and before the lesion becomes an actual invasive carcinoma. There is good evidence to indicate that this lesion does progress to invasive carcinoma if allowed to remain.

The diagnosis is almost always made by a routine Papanicolaou smear and cervical biopsy or conization of the cervix.

Treatment involves removal of the lesion. The type of procedure employed to remove the lesion frequently depends upon the age of the patient and her desire for future pregnancy. In a young patient desiring more children, removal of the entire lesion by cervical conization is accomplished. The patient is then examined frequently and cytosmears must be prepared at least every six months. In older women or those who have completed their family, abdominal or vaginal complete hysterectomy is the treatment of choice.

Invasive carcinoma. Invasive squamous cell carcinoma or adenocarcinoma of the cervix is unequivocally malignant carcinoma that has definitely invaded the stroma and, if untreated, will kill the patient (Fig. 15).

Slight intermenstrual spotting or, particularly, postcoital contact bleeding is the most frequent and usually the first symptom of carcinoma of the cervix. Spotting may be present for a short period and then not recur for two or three months. Symptoms of continuous bleeding or hemorrhaging may also occur. Leukorrhea is consistently present but is such a common symptom in women who do not have

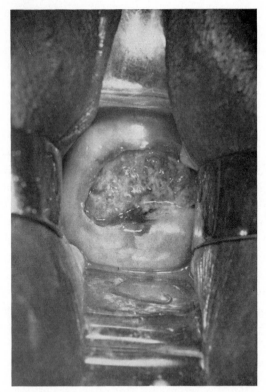

Fig. 15. Squamous cell carcinoma of the cervix.

carcinoma that its significance is hard to evaluate. Pain is usually a result of complications rather than of the disease itself unless the disease is far advanced.

The extent and stage of the lesion are based on the physical examination, which essentially determines to what extent the tumor has grown and spread within the pelvis. Clinical staging is expressed in terms of the classification of the International Federation of Gynecology and Obstetrics.

Stage   0 Carcinoma in situ.
Stage   I The carcinoma is strictly confined to the cervix.
Stage   II The carcinoma extends beyond the cervix but has not yet reached the pelvic wall; it involves the vagina, with the exception of the lower third.
Stage III The carcinoma has extended to the pelvic wall; the tumor involves the lower third of the vagina.
Stage IV The carcinoma has extended beyond the true pelvis or has involved the mucosa of the bladder or rectum.

This classification is based on the mode of spread of the tumor. This may be by direct extension to the parametrial tissue or by way of lymphatics to the lymph nodes on the lateral pelvic wall. It may also extend forward to the bladder and downward to the vaginal wall and posterior to the rectum. Classifying the lesion and knowing its mode of spread are essential in planning the course of treatment and understanding the posttherapy period.

The most common cellular type of carcinoma of the cervix is squamous cell (95%), although glandular or adenocarcinoma does occur (5%).

Radium and x-ray therapy. Treatment of carcinoma of the cervix with radiation is considered the best therapy, although some gynecologists advocate surgical procedures and others recommend radiation followed by operation. However, by far the majority of patients are treated by radium and x-ray therapy.

Radium insertion into the cervical canal and vagina plus x-ray therapy is the most frequent form of treatment used. The radium is inserted directly into the uterine cavity and is also applied externally in the vaginal vault on either side of the cervix (Fig. 16). External radiation is then administered. The object of the combined therapy is to destroy the tumor and at the same time to keep the dose of radiation within the tolerance of the normal tissues in the region. The tissue tolerance of normal structures limits the amount of radiation that can be given. Since it has been found that a large amount of radiation for a short time produces more irreparable damage than smaller amounts given over a longer period of time (protraction), radium is usually inserted in relatively low doses for a longer period of time. It is then removed and the treatment is repeated at a later date. This gives the normal cells in surrounding tissue a chance to recover from the insults of the radiation, and thus the possibility of harmful side effects is decreased. Since radium

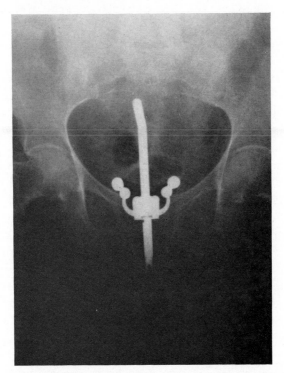

Fig. 16. Pelvic x-ray of a patient with carcinoma of the cervix, showing radium applicators in position in the uterus and vagina.

remains in the patient for several hours up to two days, the nursing-medical personnel should be well acquainted with the necessary care extended the patient in whom radium is placed and with the hazards of radiation therapy, both to the patient and to themselves.

Radium therapy. Gynecologic treatment at the present time consists of radium or cobalt. They are inserted directly into the uterine cavity with an applicator which also has ovoids for vaginal fornices radiation. By use of needles, wires, or seeds, these materials can also be inserted directly in the tissues (interstitial) involved.

In any radioactive substance a constant amount of atoms decay or disintegrate within a specific time span. The length of time necessary for the disintegration or decay of one half of the number of atoms in a certain amount (by weight) of a radioactive substance is referred to as the half-life of that substance. When a radioactive substance has a *short* half-life, it means that the amount of radioactivity decreases or decays within a short period of time, usually expressed in hours or days. Thus the exposure of the nurse to the patient receiving a short half-life radioactive substance may safely increase day by day, depending on the radioactive substance involved. If, for example, radioactive gold were involved, one half of its atoms (and activity) would be dissipated in two and one-half days. In five days only one fourth of its activity would remain. Nursing interaction with the patient would therefore change according to the *kind* of radioactive substance used in therapy and the known half-life of that substance. It would also be governed by the *amount* of the radioactive substance used and its site or method of implantation.

Radium has a long half-life of about 1,600 years. This means therefore that for this radioactive substance no decay or decrease in activity is measurable within the short time span of therapy. Because of this, nursing vigilance and restrictive precautions remain the same from the day of insertion until the careful removal of the materials and proper disposition of the radium are accomplished.

Shielding, time, and distance are considered the watchwords of protection for personnel with patients receiving radioactive substances.

Shielding means the protection of an individual from gamma or beta rays by means of mechanical shields. Gamma rays emitted by radium, radon, cobalt, and roentgen rays are effectively shielded by lead containers, applicators, aprons, or walls. Beta rays emitted by all radioactive isotopes are shielded by lead, lucite, and the density of the body tissues themselves.

Time refers to the clock time exposure of radiation to personnel in relation to the amount of radioactive substance used.

Distance refers to the rule that radiation exposure decreases proportionately as the square of the distance from the radiation increases. An understanding of this factor assists the nurse as she moves about or stands within the patient's room. It is also necessary for her to understand this as she explains to and guides the patient's relatives during this period. Evaluation and supervision of the shielding, time, and distance factors are usually responsibilities assumed by experienced nursing personnel for visitor safety.

These principles are summarized in the precautionary rules itemized by one hospital for the use of all personnel (Fig. 17).

NURSING CARE FOR PATIENTS CONTAINING INTERSTITIAL OR INTRACAVITY RADIUM, RADON OR COBALT-60

1. Every patient receiving the above treatment is to BE RESTRICTED TO BED, or placed in a private room, and SHOULD NOT BE ALLOWED TO ROAM THEREFROM during the administration of the treatment.

2. Nurses may spend whatever time is necessary near the patient for ordinary nursing care, unless Special Instructions are noted below. Private duty nurses remaining in the patients room should remain as far distant as convenient from the patient except when doing actual nursing operations.

3. Patients are allowed visitors in accordance with the usual hospital rules unless Special Instructions are given below. They should sit at least three feet from the patient.

4. Instruments and containers used to handle radium or cobalt do not themselves become radioactive and no precautions need be taken with respect to them.

5. No special precautions are needed for sputum, urine, vomitus, feces, dishes, instruments, utensils or bedding.

6. Surgical dressings and bandages should be changed only as directed by the physician in charge.

7. In Gyne cases, perineal care is not given during treatment. The pad should not be changed except under instruction from the physician in charge.

8. IF RADIUM OR COBALT NEEDLES, CONTAINERS OR CAPSULES BECOME LOOSE OR FALL OUT OR ARE REMOVED BY THE PATIENT, *DO NOT TRY TO REPLACE THEM.* CALL THE PHYSICIAN IN CHARGE IMMEDIATELY.

SPECIAL INSTRUCTIONS:

Patient's Name _____ Ward _____

This patient has inserted in _____
(Part of Body)

the following source(s) _____ *a total of*
(Needles, Tubes, etc.)

_____mc. of _____ *inserted on*
(Radium, Radon, Cobalt-60, etc.)

_____ 19 _____. To be removed on _____ 19 _____.

_____ **M.D.**

Fig. 17. Reminders for the care of patients receiving radium. (Courtesy Passavant Memorial Hospital, Chicago, Ill.)

Signs indicating radioactive therapy are placed on the door of the patient's room to remind all personnel of the special precautions required within the room or to bar the admission of certain auxiliary or housekeeping personnel. Frequent interpretation to the latter personnel will enable them to feel safe to continue communication with this patient from the door's distance, thereby minimizing the patient's degree of isolation.

THE PATIENT RECEIVING TREATMENT. The patient herself experiences a definite sense of isolation. She not only has the isolating factors of illness and pain but also the physical isolation imposed by radiation therapy. The quantity and frequency of communication between the patient and her family and the patient and the hospital personnel are greatly decreased.

The quality of the communication that does occur tends to be impersonal, objective, and even stilted when isolation conditions exist between the patient and her communicants. Thus the patient not only experiences illness, pain, and physical isolation, but in addition communication lags or breaks completely. Many observers in hospitals have surmised that the patient derives very positive benefits from her personal interactions with housekeeping and dietary personnel. However, the patient receiving radiation therapy is even denied this interest and comfort.

It is usually considered advantageous for the patient to lie flat and change position by rolling from side to side to prevent changing the position of the radium insert in any way. This means that it is difficult for the patient to eat without basic assistance, to bathe without assistance, and to cleanse herself in the genital and rectal area without assistance and it is impossible to read or write with comfort.

The radium carrier, a lead box, should be kept within the patient's room. In the event that the radioactive material is found in the bed or bedpan, it should be placed in the special box immediately, using the carrying forceps provided. It should never be handled with bare hands. All linens should be inspected carefully to make sure radium is not lost within it.

The effects of radiation therapy are directed toward destruction of abnormal tissue, sealing lymphatics, and augmenting normal tissue responses to the tumor. This means that this patient has protein loss or catabolism and may be in negative nitrogen balance. As with the operative patient, weight loss occurs and dietary intake is important to supplant the diminishing carbohydrate reserves and continuing protein losses. The frequent nausea and vomiting associated with radiation therapy often thwart the best efforts to provide varied and attractive food to this patient. Antinausea medications and tranquilizers may assist the patient over the difficult period when she needs food but cannot tolerate it. Small and frequent meals are often successful.

The patient has other problems when she is receiving radiation therapy. As with many other carcinoma patients, the gynecologic patient with carcinoma suffers the sensory insult and embarrassment of a foul odor from the disease. This may be further accentuated by the effects of the radiation process itself and by the accumulation of old blood behind the packing or applicator. Room deodorants and improved air circulation help the patient and her family with this problem.

Efforts are made to minimize the amount of sigmoid distention and thereby increase the distance between the bowel and the radioactive material. Enemas before insertion and a low fiber content diet usually achieve this objective. The patient may be given mineral oil by mouth or a small mineral oil retention enema for ease of elimination. The frequency and amount of elimination should be known for each patient in order to determine the presence of fecal material in the descending colon and rectum without the ability to defecate.

Radium therapy may produce slough of normal tissue and hemorrhage, or fistulas between the bladder and vagina and the rectum and vagina may occur. Stricture of the vagina and vault by adhesions may occur several months after the treatment.

The patient who is receiving radiation therapy has an indwelling Foley catheter in order to ensure an empty bladder at all times. If the bladder does not drain properly, the distended organ may be damaged by the radiation therapy, since the radium in the uterus is in close proximity to it. A patent catheter and tubing is therefore very necessary for this patient. Frequent observation of the drainage is required.

Any woman with an indwelling catheter feels soiled if the genitalia are not cleaned or perineal care is not given. This is especially true of the patient with radium therapy. However, hospital personnel often urge that this patient be on partial self-care. This means that if the genitalia are to be cleansed the procedure must be performed by the patient herself. This is fearful for the patient to contemplate. Yet she feels uncomfortably soiled. Fear also exists when she is required to cleanse herself after bowel elimination. If the patient is elderly or debilitated and is unable to do this for herself, a fear component arises in the nurse. How safe is it for her hands to be this close to the area of radium insertion?

PROTECTION OF PERSONNEL. Radiation from radioactive materials such as radium or radon or radioactive materials artificially produced (radioisotopes) and roentgen rays can be neither felt nor seen. Fears exist about exposure levels. Protective levels of exposure for anyone in contact with radiation have been set by the National Committee on Radiation Protection. They recommend that no personnel be exposed to greater than 5,000 milliroentgens per year and no greater than 3,000 milliroentgens within a consecutive 13-week span. In order to measure the accumulating exposure and thereby protect personnel from overexposure, many hospitals utilize film badges. These are photographic films that are sensitive to radiation exposure. All personnel assigned to the care of patients receiving radioactive therapy are given a numbered film badge that is worn at all times of personnel-patient contact. At the end of a prescribed period, usually a week, each badge is evaluated for the amount of radiation exposure to which its owner was exposed. An accumulative record is maintained for each person's exposure level. If the badge shows its wearer has been exposed to a higher accumulative record than recommended, a change in assignment is indicated for a short period of time.

Personnel who wear film badges have an assurance that their welfare is being supervised. They also feel a sense of responsibility for their own safety inasmuch as a tangible indicator of their cautious care of the patient is the film badge when it is periodically read by qualified radiologists.

That many nurses feel apprehensive of their safety when caring for the radiation patient has been found in a preliminary study. A pilot survey of six large hospitals in the Chicago area* sought the feelings of graduate nurses toward the gynecologic patient receiving radiation therapy. Question: "What do you feel are nurses' reactions to gynecologic patients receiving radioactive therapy?" Of the 51 nurses participating, 34 or 68% indicated *fear* of this patient.† Fear concerned "overexposure" and "sterility." One nurse stated, "Sometimes they [nurses] are more fearful of the radioactivity than they are concerned for the patient's needs." This fear is manifest by a "reluctance to answer the patient's light." One nurse stated, "It appears to me that the practical nurse is called upon to do those tasks that require more prolonged periods of exposure with the radium patients, in spite of the R.N.'s availability." Ten of these nurses stated that fear was minimized when proper education was extended to nurses "assigned" to such patients. A typical statement was: "Nurses who have been educated, either formally or through careful experience, react without fear in caring for patients receiving radioactive therapy." They are also assured by a knowledge of careful adherence to safety precautions by all members of the hospital staff. Nurses are able to help the patient only when all members are knowledgeable of the differences in radioactive materials, their inherent dangers, and the precautionary measures to be observed by all personnel. Education is the only true answer to any fear.

Sometimes a reevaluation of the organizational abilities and manual dexterity of the nurse will successfully help her to improve deftness and ease in giving nursing care and decrease the time required for physical care to the patient. Skilled organization and administration of nursing care proportionately minimize the exposure of personnel to radiation. The most *skilled* as well as the most *sensitive* nurse should be assigned to the care of the patient in radioactive isolation. Within a short time span she must be able to create physical comfort for a patient usually physically very uncomfortable and to convey her understanding and concern to this isolated patient.

X-ray therapy. X-ray therapy involves the patient in another isolating situation. Lying quietly for periods of time that seem very long to her, she is completely

---

*A pilot study by the authors in 1963 involved voluntary participation by graduate registered nurses (N = 51) in segregated gynecology departments or in the surgical area to which the largest number of gynecologic patients were admitted. Participating hospitals were University of Chicago Lying-In Hospitals, University of Illinois Research and Educational Hospitals, Mercy Hospital, Passavant Memorial Hospital, Wesley Memorial Hospital (all in Chicago, Ill.), and St. Francis Hospital, Evanston, Ill.

†The remaining respondents (N = 11) stated that the patient receiving radiation therapy was the "same" as any other patient. Six respondents did not answer the question.

alone with her fears and hopes for the treatment itself and for the future. All nurses caring for the patient should have communication with the personnel in the x-ray department, should know them and the environment, and should share with them verbally any information that may be pertinent to the patient's care while in x-ray therapy.

The skin of the patient receiving x-ray therapy is very sensitive because of damage to the epithelial structure. Itching is frequent, although the patient may also experience burning sharp pain. Redness and dryness of the skin are usual. Emollients may be used to alleviate this. Anything that causes further skin irritation or drying should be avoided for these patients: soap, often water, alcohol rubs, rough seams in a gown, or irritating sheets. The skin should be considered pathologic skin; therefore, external heat or cold should not be applied.

Nausea and emesis are also associated with x-ray therapy. This problem may be managed in the same ways as found advantageous when nausea existed during the period of radium therapy. Sometimes the patient finds that dry breakfast foods are easily eaten between meals and permit later foods to be eaten with decreasing nausea.

These are very uncomfortable patients whose therapy has been very extensive and who have been insulted with many stresses. They require the full extension of others who care so that their resources for sustaining and restoring themselves will not be depleted. They are often discouraged.

Carcinoma of endometrium

Adenocarcinoma of the endometrium is a disease occurring in later life (ages 40 to 60 years) and has as its most frequent symptom abnormal uterine bleeding. Postmenopausal bleeding is especially significant. Other symptoms are intermenstrual bleeding and occasionally a watery discharge. At Passavant Memorial Hospital in Chicago Wheelock* has found that the endometrial and cervical carcinomas appear in almost equal number. This is in contrast to the previously reported ratio of a one to eight incidence of endometrial to cervical carcinoma. This could be due to the fact that patients are living longer and also that there is an increased diagnostic awareness of carcinoma with postmenopausal bleeding. Fortunately, this lesion is usually slowly progressive and tends to remain localized in the uterus for a longer period of time than does carcinoma of the cervix.

Diagnostic curettage and microscopic examination of the tissue obtained are essential for diagnosis. Every patient with abnormal bleeding should be thoroughly examined. Abnormal bleeding, climacteric or postmenopausal, is considered suspicious of carcinoma until proved otherwise.

The essential treatment of carcinoma of the endometrium is surgical (Fig. 18). It is believed that an operation combined with radiation is the preferable form of therapy. Although there is no universal agreement concerning the best method of application of the radium or even whether it should be used at all, the intrauterine

---

*Wheelock, Mark: Personal communication, 1965.

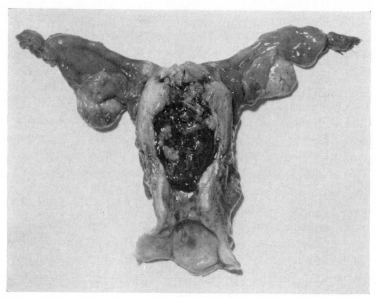

Fig. 18. Adenocarcinoma of the endometrium may be seen in the opened uterus. Both tubes and ovaries, the cervix, and the upper portion of the vagina were also removed.

application in small capsules that fill the uterus is preferred. This is followed several weeks later by a total abdominal hysterectomy and bilateral salpingo-oophorectomy. Specific contraindications to the use of radium are the presence of ovarian tumors, large fibroids, adhesions, or infection. If these are present in a patient, the pre-operative radiation is omitted. Radiation alone may be used if there is an absolute contraindication to operation. With radium in place, the previously noted radium precautions are essential (Fig. 17). The previously discussed responses of the patient during this form of therapy also pertain.

When total therapy involves radiation plus an operative procedure a few weeks later, the patient should be understood and recognized by the nursing personnel as one who not only has a serious illness but who has also had two operative insults within a short time span. Emotionally as well as physically she may be very fatigued. Her stress reserve may be low and she may remain in negative nitrogen balance for a longer period. She may be more discouraged or seem more dependent than many patients who have had only a hysterectomy. Her evidences of dependency will diminish as she feels and sees encouraging signs that she can cope with and handle this stress-laden period.

The data of the results of therapy in carcinoma of the endometrium reveals that the mortality rate is much less than that of carcinoma of the cervix. An 86% five-year survival rate has been reported. The operation of total hysterectomy and bilateral salpingo-oophorectomy is not the extensive radical operation used for carcinoma of the cervix and therefore these patients have fewer physical complications.

Carcinoma of uterine tube

Carcinoma of the uterine tube is an extremely rare lesion. The only symptoms are usually either hemorrhage, abnormal bleeding, or an abnormal gush of fluid from the vagina. Often the patient is asymptomatic. Upon physical examination a mass may be felt that cannot be distinguished from inflammatory masses of the tube. In fact the diagnosis is seldom made prior to operation. The treatment consists of surgical removal of the uterus, tubes, and ovaries. Unfortunately, the disease is usually well advanced before any symptoms are present and therefore surgical results are very poor.

Carcinoma of ovary

Carcinoma of the ovary most frequently arises in serous or pseudomucinous cystadenomas, particularly the papillary form. Malignant changes in a dermoid cyst usually consist of squamous cell carcinoma. Adenocarcinoma may arise in an endometrial cyst. Solid primary carcinoma is usually an adenocarcinoma arising from within the ovarian tissue (Fig. 19).

Metastatic carcinomas or secondary ovarian carcinomas are usually solid bilateral tumors. The primary focus is usually the endometrium, the gastrointestinal tract, or the breast. When carcinoma of the ovary is suspected, diagnostic procedures to rule out a primary source should be carried out. These include complete physical examination, curettage, and chest and gastrointestinal x-ray examinations.

Solid cancers of the ovary are much less frequent than cystic carcinomas. Approximately 50% of ovarian carcinomas are bilateral. It has been estimated by Randall* that 14 in 1,000 women over 50 years of age will develop an ovarian neoplasm and that in 8 of the 14 it will be malignant. An ovarian tumor is strongly suggestive of malignancy in women over the age of 50 years.

With malignant tumors, bilateral removal of the tubes and ovaries together with total hysterectomy is performed. In addition, omentectomy, x-ray therapy, and chemotherapy are often used as adjuncts.

Trophoblastic diseases

Hydatid mole, chorioadenoma destruens, and choriocarcinoma are tumors of the trophoblast (placenta). These tumors, which are composed of both syncytio- and cytotrophoblast, secrete chorionic gonadotropin in great amounts, estrogen, and progesterone. Accurate assay of chorionic gonadotropic hormone is indispensable in diagnosis, treatment, and follow-up of these patients. Treatment of hydatid mole is curettage, whereas in chorioadenoma and choriocarcinoma the main treatment is chemotherapy. It is in these latter trophoblastic diseases that modern research into chemotherapeutic drugs has produced results that have not been possible to obtain in any other form of cancer.

---

*Randall, C. L.: The risk of gynecologic malignancies in older women, Clinical Obstetrics and Gynecology **7:**545-555, 1964.

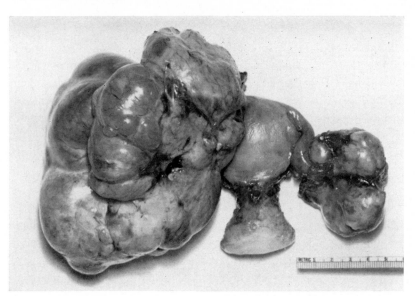

Fig. 19. A large cystic carcinoma of the ovary. It involves both ovaries.

These tumors occur more frequently in Asia, Mexico, and Africa than in the United States. In the United States there is a ratio of 1 hydatid mole to 2,500 intrauterine pregnancies, whereas in Asia the ratio is 1 to 250. Choriocarcinoma occurs in one in 40,000 to 70,000 pregnancies in the United States and in one in 250 to 4,000 in Asia.

Hydatid mole is a benign lesion in which the chorionic (placental) villi are swollen and cystic and look like small white grapes. Microscopically, there is an overgrowth of trophoblast and an absence of blood vessels in these grapelike structures. Occasionally they penetrate the wall of the uterus and may even cause uterine rupture, with hemorrhage and death, or may spread to other parts of the body without actually being a true choriocarcinoma. *Chorioadenoma destruens* or invasive mole is the term that designates this type of tumor.

Choriocarcinoma, which is one of the most malignant of all tumors, usually develops subsequent to a hydatid mole (39.2%), abortion (37.8%), or term pregnancy (23%), and rarely it is part of a teratoid tumor of the ovary. The tumor is characterized by malignant trophoblast, hemorrhage, and necrosis of tissue. Blood vessel and uterine invasion is the rule, with early metastases to the lung, vagina, brain, liver, and other organs.

Bleeding is the characteristic symptom of hydatid mole. It may be either spotting or profuse hemorrhage and occurs during the second to fourth month of pregnancy. Upon examination the uterus is larger than expected for the stage of pregnancy, and there are no positive signs of a fetus, as can be determined by fetal heart tones, fetal electrocardiograms, or x-ray visualization. Bilaterally large cystic ovaries (theca-lutein cysts) are present in 10% of the patients. Since 40% of the choriocarcinomas have been preceded by hydatid moles, it is essential that patients who have had molar pregnancies have frequent physical and x-ray examinations and, most important, chorionic gonadotropin titer assays for a period of at least two years. Abnormal bleeding, positive pregnancy tests, or metastatic lesions seen on the chest x-ray film indicate the possibility of choriocarcinoma.

The greatest pitfall in the management and treatment of these patients is the test for hormone titer. The usually employed biologic pregnancy tests have been shown to be grossly inaccurate. The bioassay method in which the mouse uterine weight is employed is essential for accurate evaluation and treatment of these patients.

Since it has been shown that trophoblastic tissue has a higher folic acid requirement than normal tissue, giving an antifolic acid compound could destroy the tumor tissue without producing irreversible toxicity in normal tissues. The primary form of therapy is the administration of methotrexate (4-amino-10-methopteroglutamic acid) which is a folic acid antagonist. Other drugs used are actinomycin-D, which is an antibiotic having an antitumor effect, and chlorambucil, which is a nitrogen mustard–alkalating agent. These drugs are given in five-day courses and repeated approximately every two weeks. Maximum effect is expected in seven days and the toxic response should occur in three to five days. The criterion for response to therapy is the chorionic gonadotropin titers ascertained seven days after treatment. Repeat examinations and serial chest x-ray examinations also provide evidence of response to treatment.

The toxic reactions to the drugs include severe stomatitis, drug rash, nausea, anorexia, and alopecia to the point of baldness. These manifestations may be treated with local analgesics, mouthwashes, and systemic analgesics if necessary. Most of these patients wear wigs, dictated by necessity and not by fashion. Daily evaluation of the patient is essential. Treatment is withheld if there is severe bone marrow depression or other toxic manifestations.

There is usually a prompt and progressive drop in the hormone titer followed by progressive regression of the metastatic lesions (usually pulmonary). Complete remission is indicated by persistent hormone titers that are normal. A later elevation of the titer in the absence of a normal pregnancy indicates recurrence of disease and therapy is reinstituted.

If resistance to methotrexate becomes apparent, the other drugs, actinomycin-D and chlorambucil, are given.

In an effort to retain the reproductive capacity of young women with trophoblastic disease, a new group of patients is being studied from the standpoint of chemoprophylaxis. Using chemotherapy alone, the results have been most encouraging and some women with malignant trophoblastic disease have had subsequent normal pregnancies. Thus, in this area of cancer, research has proved to be most beneficial, with actual cures possible.

Formerly it was believed that patients with choriocarcinoma treated surgically seldom survived; and if the patient did survive, the diagnosis was considered incorrect. This idea has been dispelled by Brewer,* who reported that the absolute five-year survival rate of 122 patients treated by hysterectomy was 31.9%; if metastases were present at the time of hysterectomy, the survival rate was 19.2%. Although these figures are much better than had been generally taught, they do not approach the favorable results reported by both the National Institutes of Health and by the Northwestern University group, who have obtained a 48 to 55% survival rate in patients with metastatic trophoblastic disease treated with chemotherapy.*

These patients all know they have a malignancy. When told of the character of this disease, their anxiety mounts and the fear of pain, mutilation, and death is great. They are young women who have young growing families at home, often a young infant. Their worries are for them and for themselves. The individual toxic reactions to the therapy itself are frightening and discouraging. Apart from the esthetic quality, hair has other connotations to the woman. Its loss provokes a severe emotional reaction. The presence of nausea and often coexistent stomatitis presents a challenge to the ingenuity of both the nurse and dietitian.

The presence of all toxic responses means that the patient receiving therapy faces the reality that she must "get worse" before she "gets better." This is also difficult for the members of the helping-healing professions to cope with. Doctor, patient, and nurse have always been bound in the common experience of therapeutic uncertainty or assurance. Recent research gives increasing credence to the beneficial effects of therapy extended with the faith and conviction of the doctor and the nursing staff. Therapy extended with uncertainty is uncertain. These patients require frequent contact with the helping-healing professions who believe in the therapeutic plan, who understand and recognize the daily discomforts and accumulating discouragements, stresses, and vicissitudes that the therapy imposes, and who believe in the cooperative and interdependent nature of the helping-healing process with the patient.

THE PATIENT'S KNOWLEDGE OF HER DISEASE

The patient with carcinoma exemplifies the degree of patient isolation created and permitted when few if any of her personal contacts are willing to share with her the feelings of life's tenacity and to help her in her valley of the shadow.

The perennially plaguing question, "Should the patient be told the truth?" really involves personal answers to even more basic and unacknowledged questions. These originate as, "How will *I* feel telling her?" "How should I tell her?" and "Would I be able [be willing] to sustain and help her with the amount of help she will require *after* she knows the truth?"

It is often stated: "The patient will ask when she wants to know." *Whom* she asks will depend on the kind of personal interaction she has had with individuals

---

*Brewer, John I., et al.: Chemotherapy in trophoblastic diseases, American Journal of Obstetrics and Gynecology **90:**566, 1964.

in the helping professions. A relationship may have existed prior to operation and immediately thereafter that discouraged the patient from asking questions of any kind. *When* she can ask is also dependent on the actions of others. An authoritarian relationship or repeated experiences with the doctor or nurse when time pressures severely influence communication will also influence the ability and willingness of the patient to ask the nature of her illness and its treatment. Repeated sidestepping of the answers sought or unintelligible answers to the patient will discourage her from repeated questioning. No one continues to ask for help when help is grudgingly or insufficiently given. No one can be insensitive to a denied request for help. The unanswered question, the ignored question, the sidestepped question by responding, "ask the doctor that question," or an insincere assurance that "everything will be all right," are denials of help to the patient. The refusal to help and to "level" with the patient leaves her alone, uncertain of her situation, and therefore unassisted in maintaining and implementing necessary adaptive armamentarium to cope with the existing and long-term incapacitation.

To recognize a patient as an individual who possesses self-worth and dignity also implies a recognition of that individual's potentials for personal growth and her continuing ability to cope with an ever-changing world. Helping the patient to help herself within a difficult period enhances the stature of that individual and encourages personal growth, even in the presence of physical decline. Judging the individual incapable or too weak to participate in her own life's work is to *devalue* her and to deny the efficiency of her coping mechanisms to tolerate change. Her weakness is identified; her strength is ignored. The often quoted example of the "weak individual" who could not "take the news" is usually one to whom a flat pronouncement of doom was made and no further help extended to assist her in handling a totally new life situation and a nebulous future.

Perhaps there *are* unique patients whose previous instability in life crises has been known. Even so, the settings and meanings of each crisis to an individual make each crisis different. Even they cannot be generalized. Perhaps there are *some* patients who cannot handle the terminal period of their life. However, when this judgment is *made for* most or all patients, discomfort, uneasiness, and fear of life's end may be identified in those making that judgment.

For most patients the insincere game played by her family, friends, and the trusted professions may devitalize the patient's confidence in everything they now say to her. Patient and family may be separated by a gulf of distrust, guilt, hurt, and discomfort in one another's presence. Whether verbally communicated or not, the patient sooner or later "knows" she has a fatal illness. If she cannot speak of this to anyone because of their refusal to admit the truth to her or because of their discomfort and their adherence to "the game," she must be isolated and unable to share with anyone her thoughts of separation, her grief, and her mounting and changing needs for emotional and spiritual strength. Does this not compound a situation already identified as too stressful and traumatic for the patient to tolerate? If she is stable enough to cope with the situation all alone, would she not also have been able to hear the truth of her condition? Could she not have better adjusted her life with the extended love and understanding of her family and the helping professions throughout the period than to be ostracized from those who could have helped? During the period of grief after the death of a loved one, the immediate mourners usually *want* to talk of the death and the loved one. The intermediate mourners and acquaintances often find this uncomfortable and embarrassing. Do the conversation and the questioning of the patient who does know the truth make us feel uneasy, uncomfortable, and helpless? Is this sometimes the reason why a patient is not told about her illness?

The individual nurse's personal philosophy of life, sickness, and death will influence her answer to this question and her relationship with this patient. Her feelings toward medical science and her role in it will also influence her answer and her relationship with this patient. If, for example, the nurse feels a strong partner relationship with the doctor and potential mastery over disease for the patient, she may experience defeat and depression or anger in the face of unsuccessful therapy and ensuing terminal illness. She may find it very difficult to talk and spend time with the patient who is the symbol of a medical failure.

The nurse who sees her role within a helping profession as being interdependent with all the helping professions *with* the patient will not feel personal defeat but intensified concern for the individual within a difficult situation who requires her sensitivity, understanding, and giving in a new way and in greater measure. Through this emphasis the mother and wife may be helped and sustained so that she in turn may feel capable of setting her physical and spiritual house in order. The patient may wish to prepare her children in many individual ways during this period. She may indeed provide many strengths to her family. Her ability to give to them, however, may be dependent on someone in the helping professions sustaining (giving to) her throughout the period.

During this period when the duration of personal contacts is unknown to the patient, the numbers of these contacts should not diminish, especially those that mean understanding and stability to her. For this reason, contact with the helping professions is necessary. Periodic contact with the doctor by phone or office visits is necessary to her, even though no new hopes can be expected or extended. Periodic visits by the public health nurse (even when little or no physical care is necessary) often provide a necessary and secure contact.

It may be considered wise to advise seeking the help of a homemaker or another adult member of the family so that physically exhausting home responsibilities may be relieved and the patient's time and energies may be extended to her husband and children. When the nurse is interested in the wisest investment of the future for the individual patient, she can be the instrument that makes possible a home evaluation and realistic home plans for the patient. She can be the person to counsel the family for future sources of help.

Local offices of the American Cancer Society vary in their ability to furnish transportation to the patient requiring daily therapy or to make available the varying contents of their loan closets. These and other community resources available for this patient should be known by the hospital and office nurse, not only by the public health nurse.

When "the game" of "let's pretend there's nothing wrong" is played with the patient and her family, many forms of assistance can never be extended to the patient to lighten the difficulties of the period. She is forced to walk alone because she is too weak to be helped by the "strong."

THE EFFECT OF "CANCER" ON OTHERS

The fears of hereditary transmission and the contagious transmission of "killer" diseases have long existed. The question of transmissibility often arises within the family or close friends of a patient with terminal "cancer." Because of their personal involvement with the patient, the question is often denied or ignored. However, many patients feel the effects of their relatives' fears. Dishes, linen, and even the patient herself may be isolated from the family's contact.

Recent research that links a virus with cancer has had a renewed influence on the general public. Because of the visible effects of the disease and the existing uncertainty of the causal agents, the question of transmissibility now exists in many nonprofessional personnel. Fear or dread of the cancer patient by anyone "caring" for her will be reflected in the quality and quantity of "care" given to her. Fear of the patient further isolates her from those who are most capable of helping her.

When the information media of today report individual studies and preliminary findings to the general public, the meaning and significance of these research endeavors to the whole disease problem should be explained to auxiliary personnel and ancillary professions within the hospital environs. Fear is dissipated when knowledge and understanding grow. The transmissibility of cancer remains obscure. Unacknowledged but growing fear in the general population should not go unnoticed lest the cancer patient become treated as the leper of old who was required to wear a bell.

THE TERMINALLY ILL PATIENT

Delay in therapy or unresponsiveness to therapy results in metastatic carcinoma or carcinomatosis. Gynecologic malignancies extend by direct infiltration into adjacent tissues and by lymphatic and vascular metastasis (Fig. 20).

The reproductive organs of the woman are also the sites of secondary metastatic lesions. Thus secondary carcinoma of the ovary may occur when the primary site is in the gastrointestinal tract by direct extension or by blood or lymph circulations. Secondary ovarian carcinoma may have had its primary foci in the breast. Secondary malignancies of the cervix and tube are not common. When they occur, they are usually due to a direct extension from adjacent tissue rather than a distant metastatic site. Secondary adenocarcinoma may originate as a primary lesion in the breast, gastrointestinal tract or ovary.

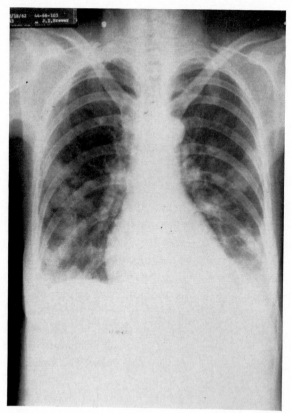

Fig. 20. Chest x-ray film, showing multiple pulmonary metastases of choriocarcinoma.

Since many tissues and many metastatic sites may be involved in any patient, the nurse does not extend nursing care to the gynecologic patient but to a patient with a malignant disease that influences many systems and organs. She must be ever cognizant of the importance of astute observations and evaluations of the patient's condition from one period of contact to another. Changes in elimination or urinary output, fatigue, early cough, orthopnea, presence of nodules, and new or old bleeding are pertinent for the reevaluation of the patient's course and the assumption of sustaining or palliative therapies. As she is horrified or sorrowed by the appearance of each new symptom, the sensitive nurse will be acutely aware of the patient's fears and anxieties at such signs. Symptoms observed in silence with no medical comment or explanation stimulate great patient and family anxiety and uncertainty, especially when present lay education emphasizes patient reporting of symptoms of bleeding, lumps, changes in elimination habits, or cough.

PAIN

Pain in the patient with carcinoma is often interrelated with the presence of anxiety and nausea. This usually means that the pain reaction is great when the latter coexist. The patient with a malignancy often requires help in interpreting the severity of her pain and the medication to use. As pain increases in severity and/or duration, she often hesitates to take increasing amounts of medication, even though the doctor's prescription order would permit her to do so. All patients are very fearful of "getting so used to a drug that it will not be effective" when they need it. They also fear addiction and often bear nights and days heavy with pain rather than take repeated doses of a narcotic prescribed for them. When so many analgesics are available today, effective pain alleviation can be attained for most patients. The medications can be rotated in use so that the prevalent fears and the actual instances of drug dependency are minimized. The patient requires and deserves a pain-free state. She also requires and deserves reassurances that she will not be addicted because the medication will be changed before that time occurs. She requires constant and careful evaluations of her pain, her reactions to it, and her medications. Because of her closeness to the patient, the hospital, office, or public health nurse is most capable of interpreting this for the doctor. The patient feels this is important to her but is of relative insignificance to the doctor. She is more inclined to discuss pain at length with the nurse. The nurse can also be the professional person most available to help the family interpret the patient's pain and to help them cope with the experience of witnessing pain in a loved one.

Pain and its language arouse feelings of uneasiness and discomfort in anyone who witnesses it in another. This feeling may extend to include sorrow and guilt in those emotionally involved with the patient. A wish to deny the presence of any of these feelings may result in new feelings of anger, impatience, or resentment directed toward pain itself and deflected or directed to the patient experiencing that pain. This may occur in anyone in contact with pain. When that pain is long term and cannot be fully alleviated, the "pain" of those witnessing it is accentuated. It is essential for the nurse to recognize her feelings in the presence of pain, how it changes with different individuals, and how she reacts or copes with her feelings. Only then can she effectively help the patient's family with their problems in the face of pain and interpret to the patient the reason for the sometimes unsympathetic attitudes of those around her. The patient is always isolated in her pain. She can be helped by those who try to understand it and who try to alleviate that isolation by minimizing the patient's distance from others.

When terminal care is necessary, the patient and family again require the understanding and guidance of the helping professions. Often symptoms occur that are remote from the site of the original operation and may remain obscure unless the family learns what may be anticipated and how to cope with it. They require help in physically caring for the patient and in the preparation of appetite-appealing food, which to some families becomes the last and only successful expression of giving to the patient. The sources of inexpensive or free dressings, walkers, commodes, rubber rings, sheep skins, etc. are important helps. Helpful to the patient herself and her family, they also provide future assurances to the family that they did all they could.

If the patient is depressed or irritable, or if the family is unable to handle the situation without great physical, emotional, or financial difficulty, more frequent assistance of the public health nurse, the physician, or other helping professions such as social workers are necessary.

During the past few years some prominent individuals (Eleanor Roosevelt, Gary Cooper, and Dick Powell, to name a few) have insisted on home care rather than hospitalization during the final phase of their illness. Many patients may prefer to remain within familiar comforting home surroundings and within the circle of family and friends who have given their life substance and meaning. Many families, too, may prefer to keep the mother and wife close to them. During this period they require frequent communication with the doctor, the public health nurse, or the nurse-neighbor for interpretation of the patient's condition and guidance in day-by-day care and in understanding their own reactions. Physical and emotional withdrawal from the patient in the home or hospital may occur if the family is frightened, overwhelmed, or hostile to the progressive illness state. The family and patient require help during this period.

Hospital care during the final phase of illness may relieve the family of many fearful responsibilities. The availability of medical and nursing care within the hospital and the hope that something can still be done or that the best will be done may be reassuring to some families and patients. Others may be relieved by hospitalization but may feel regret or guilt that home care was not possible or successful.

The decision for home or hospital care is an important and an individual one for every patient and her family. It is a mutual decision made by the patient, family, and helping-healing professions.

RECOMMENDED READINGS FOR STUDENTS

Abrams, Ruth D., and Finesinger, Jacob: Guilt reactions in patients with cancer, Cancer **6:** 474-482, 1953.

Cobb, Beatrix: Emotional problems of adult cancer patients, Journal of the American Geriatrics Society **7:**274-285, 1959.

Standard, Samuel, and Nathan, Helmuth, editors: Should the patient know the truth, New York, 1955, Springer Publishing Co., Inc. (A collection of essays by surgeons, internists, psychiatrists, nurses in many fields, clergy of different faiths, and lawyers.)

Sutherland, Arthur M.: The psychological impact of post-operative cancer, Bulletin of the New York Academy of Medicine **33:**428-445, 1957.

Pamphlets

A handbook on radiation for nurses, New York, no date, The Nursing Division, Memorial Hospital for Cancer and Allied Diseases, Memorial Sloan-Kettering Cancer Center.

Handbook of rules for administration of radioactive materials to patients, New York, 1959, E. R. Squibb and Sons. (Through special permission of the M. D. Anderson Hospital and Tumor Institute, Texas Medical Center, Houston, Texas.)

RECOMMENDED READINGS FOR INSTRUCTORS AND THE EXCEPTIONAL STUDENT

Brewer, John I.: Textbook of gynecology. Baltimore, 1961, The Williams & Wilkins Co.

Brewer, John I., et al.: Chemotherapy in trophoblastic diseases, American Journal of Obstetrics and Gynecology **90:**566-578, 1964.

Meerlo, Joost: Psychological implications of cancer, Geriatrics **9:**154-156, 1954.

Randall, C. L.: The risk of gynecologic malignancies in older women, Clinical Obstetrics and Gynecology **7:**545-555, 1964.

Wright, Beatrice A.: Physical disability: A psychological approach. New York, 1960, Harper & Row, Publishers, pp. 108-117.

TYPICAL READINGS ACCESSIBLE TO PATIENTS

Davis, Olive Stull: My Life with Cancer, Ladies' Home Journal **81**(9):68-69, 122, 124, 126, 1964.

Pamphlets

American Cancer Society, Inc., New York.

Index